I0455189

The Wellbeing Touch

An Uncomplicated guide to great
health - naturally!

By
Wendy Langley

Contents

Disclaimer:

This book is intended as an information and educational guide and is not a medical textbook. It is not intended to replace professional healthcare. The publisher and author are not responsible for any suggestions discussed in this book or for any reader who chooses to self-prescribe.

About me

Hi I am Wendy Langley
I am a Natural Health Specialist, Personal Trainer and
self-confessed chocoholic!
But we will talk about that later.

Like you, I am constantly doing my best to become better than I was yesterday and trying to put my stamp on the universe. Keeping in good health helps me to do that, and a whole lot more besides, and staying fit and healthy can help you do the same too!

I am living the 'dream'. It is my dream, but hey, I have got here despite the many obstacles that were placed in my way. Although my dream requires a little tweaking from time to time, I pave my own road, face my own challenges, learn my lessons, eat well, think big, have fun, laugh lots, and do my best to help others on my way.

I absolutely adore spending time with my man, hosting family days with the gang and doing coffee with friends. I have one dog and five cats who are known as 'The happy bunch'. I love eating delicious food, drinking fine wine, watching musical movies, (old and new,) dancing, laying on the beach in the sun with a good book (and the love of my life, of course!) and swimming in the crystal clear seas of Crete.

Twelve years ago, due to ill health and the stresses of life, I kissed goodbye to a dance career that spanned thirty two years. But there is a silver lining to EVERYTHING and a change bought with it a new profession. So my dance career turned to nutrition, my event staging turned to diet planning, my teaching turned to coaching and my theatre has become a book!

I am a qualified Nutritional Therapist, Life Coach, Personal Trainer, Dance Teacher, Cognitive Behavioural Therapist and Neuro Linguistic Programming Therapist, which I use in various combinations to help those I treat. I have run my own, successful Natural Health Consulting business for many years and have lots of happy, healthy clients to show for it.

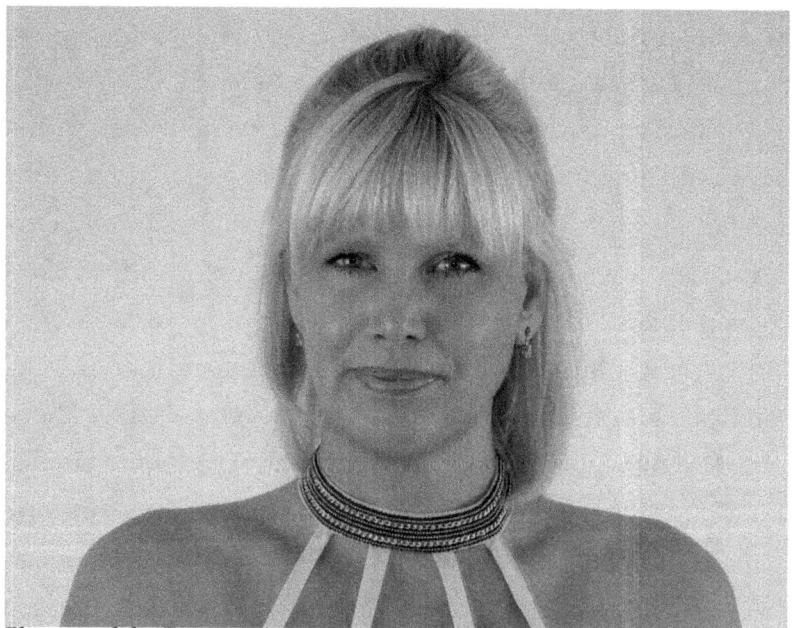

Photograph by Ramin Arbabi of http://www.winningwaysmedia.com

I don't have all the answers to all the health issues out there, and there is always plenty more for me to learn, but I am happy I am able to share with you what I have learned so far!

You are welcome to join The Wellbeing Touch Facebook page, which offers daily tips on nutrition, health, and keeping motivated. I write for the online health and wellbeing magazine, Jeunissima – the art and joy of feeling young, a great publication that's worth a read and, if that is not enough, The Wellbeing Touch website includes a wealth of health information including The Tasting Plate, an ever-growing collection of tasty and health boosting recipes.

But, if you are constantly battling your health or your life, then perhaps we need to consult over a coffee - real or virtual - pronto!

Website: www.thewellbeingtouch.com

Let's make an introduction

"May you live every day of your life."
— Jonathan Swift

Welcome to The Wellbeing Touch –an uncomplicated guide to great health….naturally. What is it about? It is an easy going read about having fabulous health the natural way, through the foods you eat, exercise, your attitude to life, and a little supplementation. Being fit and healthy is my passion as well as my own personal journey, so I welcome you to join in, reap the benefits and never look back my friend.

For the last twelve years I have been working to perfect my own health using natural means and, in my current role as a Natural Health Practitioner, I help numerous others to do the same. It all came about when the conventional medicine path let me down and I was left in a very poor state of health mentally and physically. Ill health cost me my career, my relationship at the time, and turned my world upside down. It was not a good time in my life and I needed to 'do or die'. Fortunately, my friend, I am not one to lie down and give up, so I stepped up, took control, and decided to do, certainly not die!

With anything you do, if you over indulge you tend to pay the price. I over indulged in a dance career and as a result I paid the price with my health. I combined excessive exercise (yes you can do too much!) with a diet suitable for an anorexic ant. This was complicated by the annual stress of pupil dance exams, shows, TV appearances, and a very challenging personal life. In reality it was my ignorance that took me down the slippery slope to ill health and it has been my education since that time that has bought me back up to where I am now.

Today I am walking proof that health can be regained and sustained using natural methods and the right mind set. Sometimes I have to re- adjust what I do and how I do it, adapting to the day by day life changes and circumstances that create changes in me. However I am thankful for the lessons life brings,(even if I do sometimes curse a little under my breath) and I am fitter, healthier and happier than I have been in years. 'Pain is temporary. Glory is forever'. And they are right!

Health, contrary to popular belief, is not just the absence of disease my friend -there is a little more to it than that. Being healthy is about having an inner energy and zest for life, both physically and mentally, that enables you to live a full and happy existence. It's like feeling it is your birthday every day! It involves a harmonious body and mind connection which in its truest sense makes health 'holistic' – encompassing the whole of you. It is about living as one with yourself, feeling content and peaceful with who you are, no matter how you are, and not being trapped in your own civil war!

Being a bit unhealthy, or becoming quite sick, does not happen by accident, or over-night, and it is the end result after your body has been telling you for some time that things are not right. You would probably have ignored the warning signs such as recurrent infections, tiredness, insomnia, irritability, low mood, fatigue or indigestion and possibly brushed them off as being part and parcel of your age.

However and whenever, your body started to be out of sync you can bet your bottom dollar it would have been screaming at you, jumping up and down and waving a red flag at you, desperately trying to get your attention. The sad thing is many of us fail to pay attention – deliberately or not. Eventually the ignored body loses the battle to get help and slips into degeneration and you end up with a state of disease – otherwise known as disease. Then you have to sit up and pay attention and so the battle to fix the problem begins. My friend, prevention is so much easier than cure and learning to listen to your body could save you a whole lot of misery and even save your life.

On the bright side, as we should always look on the bright side of life, (feel free to break into song) if you provide your body with the right conditions it will often heal itself as it will have all it needs to heal and rejuvenate, plus a very efficient immune system which is capable of seeing off any nasty invader. By taking an avid interest in yourself, giving your body the right tools and plenty of self- care your body will respond in a very positive way and do its best to keep you fit and healthy. Your body is one amazing piece of kit!

Our health is not something to take lightly, indeed we need to understand that it is our responsibility to take great care of it; but if we approach it with a sense of humour and lightness we can keep it more in perspective. We do tend to act way too seriously about so many things in life, probably because since we were young we have been told to 'Take things seriously,' or ' Be serious' or even 'Take yourself seriously.' When we act in such a way we begin to worry and stress which certainly does not help the situation or make any issue disappear. In fact stressing and worrying can make the problem so much bigger as we blow it out of all proportion, and this in itself can cause us to become sick or sicker- which is not the aim of the game! Our health is something we have control over and a choice about. So it makes sense that instead of moaning or fretting about it we should step up and do something about it instead. So, let's do exactly that!

It is not complicated to be fit and well, although the media out there causes such a lot of confusion and controversy about how we should best take care of ourselves. Keeping things simple in this life makes living a whole lot easier and a much more pleasant experience. There is no reason to become a scientist in order to know how to look after yourself and it will not cost you fortunes to do so either. I believe most people have been lead to believe that being fit and healthy is a very involved and costly procedure. Fear not, for I am here to convince you otherwise. Why would we want to make something as essential as good health complicated? My friend, let's do this the easy way. I am all for making life as easy and stress free as possible, so that we have plenty of time to kick off our shoes and enjoy it!

The Wellbeing Touch e-book is designed as an uncomplicated guide, sharing my knowledge and experiences which will hopefully help you understand how to sustain your own health a little better. It is about understanding food – your fuel for life, and adopting some uncomplicated attitudes that will help you be fit and well, as the whole person you are. There are no references to research, as I have chosen not to complicate things with scientific language and have written this book as one that is straightforward to read. These days, of course, we have the internet, stacked full of information should you choose to do some further research on any subject I have raised. Sometimes life is simpler than you think and being healthy is not a complicated art........

I wish you great health my friend and happy reading. But just in case, as you read this, you think that I have the weirdest bunch of clients ever – I have chosen to give all the client examples character names from Sesame Street, to add a little lightness to their stories. Making the reading a little fun I believe, makes the reading a little easier! It reminds me of the days when my sons were young and I used to help them read their books for school when they were bored. We used the 'sausage and mash' form of reading (I am sure this comes with the approval of the top universities!) – you know where you change every word that begins with an 's' into sausage and every word that begins with an 'm' into mash. The reading was always full of hilarity, but this way we managed to read every book they were ever asked to read. And they both finished school with fantastic grades – proof that a bit of fun makes learning a little easier!

A life time of taste.

From your Cordon Bleu restaurant, to your local take out,
Your homemade fair and smoked salmon trout
From your cakes and sweet buns, your dark chocolate treats,
To your crocodile steaks and barbequed meats,
From the orange you picked direct from the tree
To the fruity jam on your luscious cream tea.
From the puddings and pies served with mushy green peas,
To your Beoef Bourgignon with garlic green beans.
From the hollandaise eggs, with spinach below,
To the thick, crusty bread that they make from fresh dough.
From the sushi and hot dogs and sweet meringue pie,
To the beautiful wedding cake piled upon high.
From the lentils and beans for a way healthy meal
To the mussels and whelks and strange jellied eel.
From the fine lobster bisque to the pizza and chips
And those little chopped crudités sliced for the dips.
From the berries and cherries that welcome our fall
And the nuts and the seeds and the raisins and all
We all love our food, be it healthy or not
Whether cooked in a pan, on the grill, in a pot.
In a stir fry, a stew, a roast or just raw,
At a posh dinning venue or on a mat on the floor.
Our food is our fuel, our health and our life,
Be wise what you place on your fork and your knife.

9

Why go natural?

"The best and most efficient pharmacy is within your own
system."
— Robert C. Peal

When I was a child my sister and I would become
very embarrassed by a certain habit my mother had. We would
wince, pull horrified faces at each other and wish to hide. What
did my mother do to make us feel like this? She would sing out
loud whenever we were waiting for a bus! As we did not have
a car, we were frequently using buses to go on journeys of any
distance, so the singing was a regular occurrence. What made
it all slightly worse was that she never managed to recall all the
words for any one song, so there were a lot of ad libs and tra
la las thrown in. And to make things even more excruciating
the buses were notorious for being late and there was always a
queue of people…staring at us! Of course, since I, myself have
been a mother I have realised that embarrassing your children
can actually be rather a lot of fun, although I have not had the
urge to sing at bus stops - well not yet! However, it was not my
mother's intention to embarrass us, (so she says), it was just her
happy way and she loved to sing. She is incredible, really, to
be so full of joyful songs being as life has not been that easy for
her. Upon consideration I have realised it must have been down
to the naturally healthy lifestyle she unwittingly followed that
kept her in fine tune. Healthy people are happy people and

blasting out a bit of 'Happy Talk' (occasionally with actions!) at the bus stop was a sure sign that mum was in great health.

I am sure you realise that many of the chronic diseases of the West are caused by poor dietary and lifestyle choices. So it seems to make perfect sense to change the poor habits we have, in order to give us the upper hand when it comes to how well we remain fit and healthy. It's simple really -if we eat a healthy diet, exercise like we should, have a positive outlook on life and manage our stress we should be rocking (and singing) our way into the twilight years.

However, many people do not seem to appreciate the very fact that maintaining good health can be down to such simple things as eating the right food, taking a little exercise or drinking more water. Instead, when we are not feeling so great, we will more than likely reach for a pill to fix the ill! There are plenty of advertisements encouraging you to buy a potion or two to fix your complaints, usually with actors in white coats so they seem to you and I like doctors (a clever marketing ploy). Actually all these advertised lotions and potions do is treat your symptoms, not address the cause, which means you could well suffer from the same complaint on and off over a period of time. But as we have become so dependent on a 'quick fix pill' these days, why would you bother, and how are you expected to know, how you can naturally help yourself in ways other than by administering medication?!

It's hardly a secret that the more medicine we take - whether they are bought over the counter or prescribed to us by a doctor - the less likely our bodies are able to respond to it.

In deed as I am writing this, there is a whole lot of talk about antibiotics and how we need to keep finding new ones as our bodies are becoming non responsive to the antibiotics available. As we continue to take medicines, we build a tolerance to them, which means it will eventually become necessary to up the dose from one pill to two, or two spoons to three, and so on. Unfortunately there is a constant barrage in the media to treat everything from colds and flu, pain to heartburn, or even weight issues by taking some pill or another and so it's easy to see why we tend to turn immediately to medicine once something is wrong. We have become a society that looks for a 'quick pill fix'. However, if we do turn to medicinal solutions for every sniffle we get, what chance will we have of the medication working well when we really need it to?

There are numerous advertisements for one pain killer or another to combat your headache, but have you noticed there is a complete absence of advertisements informing us that the best way to get rid of a headache is to sip water throughout the day. (There is more money in encouraging you to take a pill than drink a glass of water). How many people do you think actually know that dehydration is one of the major causes of those nasty, banging headaches? Well, you, my friend, are one more now! And simply by drinking water you could banish the pain!

There are plenty of health issues that can be and would be better treated purely by adopting a healthier lifestyle my friend, rather than pursuing the easy option of the doctor's pill. In the long run medication itself will cause other health related problems, which will then need further medical treatment, until a person could eventually find that what started off as one pill a day to control one health issue, has escalated to a handful of various pills to fix a various amount of health issues! All conventional medicines are drugs and with such, come the various side effects too.

I feel it important to add here that I am not against medication, indeed medicine has made significant changes in how well we survive and it certainly has its place. It is just that we don't always need to take medicine as there are other ways to look after our health. At the end of the day medicines can weaken the body's defences and make it harder for other medicines to come to its aid, with some medicines causing enough damage, as I have said, that you may well need to take another in order to put the damage right and so on. This is all beneficial to the pharmaceutical companies, who are a multi-billion pound industry, and of course to those who promote such drugs and get paid handsomely to do so, but maybe it is not so beneficial to you.

There are many ways to treat your health naturally, without constantly turning to medicine. A natural approach may even be more effective, and at the same time, you'll be boosting your body's natural defences rather than depleting another part. Nature offers a huge medicine cabinet at our disposal, with food, herbs and spices that have been used for thousands of years to treat sickness and to encourage a strong and healthy body. It would be rude not to use these super healing nutrients when Mother Nature has left them as a gift for us. We also have super healing powers within our own hands.

Think of yourself as Superman (with or without the blue pants over your tights), or Wonder Woman (complete with fabulous outfit and figure to go in it) when it comes to your health. If we make a conscious decision to do something about our health and make simple changes and adjustments to the way we live each day, we can make vast differences in how well we are.

We all know that prevention is easier than cure on all levels. Preventing cancer, heart disease, diabetes, obesity, arthritis or even a cold, as you can well imagine, is a far kinder route than having to fight the good fight with them. Given the choice, I am sure we would all choose to live without these health issues and that is why doing our best to prevent them in the first place is one of the greatest health plans we can put in place.

Food plays an enormous role in how healthy we are and is the most natural way to ensure we live a pain free, disease free life. Exercise will enhance the benefits of good nutrition by keeping your body physically and mentally in shape. Managing your stress will give you a lighter take on life and will relieve you of the disease causing ability that stress has. Having a balanced, positive outlook on life will see it all come together beautifully and you will be dancing, and singing in the rain!

Do your best my friend to stay away from the medicine cupboard and take care of your health naturally. It is easier to do this than you might believe. A combination of healthy food choices, stress management, a positive outlook and daily exercise will have you enjoying great health. One step at a time, slowly, slowly, you can do this. Here's how.....

Where do we begin? At the very beginning, of course!

"If we are creating ourselves all the time, then it is never too late to begin creating the bodies we want instead of the ones we mistakenly assume we are stuck with."
— Deepak Chopra

It's always a great idea to start at the very beginning, so let's start from the moment you were a twinkle in your father's eye. Your health journey began before you were conceived. We have known for many years that smoking can harm an unborn child, and those who take drugs during pregnancy can have children who are drug dependent. But what about the foods your parents ate, the drink they drank and the stress they were under before and when you were conceived? Did you know that all these had an impact too? Well if you didn't before, you do now! That does not mean to say that you can blame your parents for the state of your health - only you are responsible for that - but it does mean that your start will have a bearing on your health tendencies and predisposition which is helpful to know and understand.

Parents who ate a diet high in junk food will have put their children at risk of developing a taste for junk food, with sugar being up there at the top of the addiction list. This link is now well established in scientific research. So, again, not blaming your parents, obviously, but could you have a tendency to make unhealthy food choices due to your parent's diet and lifestyle, before your birth?

If you are pregnant or planning a pregnancy it is especially vital to eat healthily to aid fertility, help your baby to develop and grow, and to keep you fit and well too. Looking after mum is of equal importance as ensuring bump grows well. There is not really the need to eat for two (or more), but there is a need to have a great variety of nutrients constantly. Supplementation is a great idea, before, during and after pregnancy to keep those necessary nutrients topped up, but it is best to take professional advice as to what is suitable.

If you believe this to be true in your case, there is no reason to continue on the same path. You have to remember that as an adult, you are responsible for your health and you have the power to change. You have choices. You can choose to be unhealthy or you can choose to be healthy. You can choose to eat healthily, or you can choose to eat unhealthily. As you have purchased this book, I will take it that you have chosen to do something about your health, which is a great start!

As a coach, it is my job to help people with the present moment and how making the most of the present (which is by its very name, a gift!), and facilitating change where necessary, they will be on the road to a glorious future. I do not concentrate on the past, because it has come and gone and we cannot change it. Of course, there is a need to take a person's past health issues into consideration, but then it is all about change...because if you do not like where you are now, you need to change things. If you do not change, then life will continue exactly as it is, which is counter-productive if you wish things to be different!

So what about when you were growing up? What were you given to eat? I grew up in a relatively poor household, but it was healthy. My mother cooked very good, old fashioned English food, always from scratch. Meals were padded out with vegetables as they were cheaper than meat. If we wanted a snack it was always an apple. We were rarely allowed sweets, only had fizzy drinks at Christmas, and an occasional ice cream soda in the then, hot summer. Crisps were a rarity, and cakes were mainly home -made when my mother had time. So we were a healthy bunch. My father was a postman, my mother a nursery school head, I danced 6 days a week , along with one sister and my other sister had riding lessons, so we were a very active family and this remains the case today!

We recently celebrated my youngest son's 18th Birthday and had a bouncy castle in the garden for the children to enjoy at the party. But bouncing and enjoying the castle was not only for the smaller members of the family. Indeed, bouncing away was I, my sister and my 79 year old mother! My 89 year old father was standing watching, laughing and taking photographic evidence! Told you we are an active bunch!

I know this is not the same story for everyone. Sadly, I believe that the younger generations today are at an even greater risk of disease because of the standard of food that is readily accessible. Although we live in a time where everyone is talking recession, money is spent on food, in particular the cheap, more convenient choices of processed foods. You will see school children piling into the 'express' supermarkets to gather their sweets, crisps and fizzy drinks, pre packed sandwiches, pies and pasties before school. As responsible parents, shouldn't we be able to educate and nurture our babies better? We would fiercely protect our children from a stranger who may be a killer, so why do we not protect them from diets that may cause cancer, diabetes, strokes and heart attacks or years of suffering from challenging weight issues?

Start your day the correct way which, my friend, is not with sugar laden cereals or toast and jam...sorry. The first thing to land in your stomach should be a good dose of quality protein – fish, eggs, meat, plain live yogurt, nuts, seeds or even a 'good' protein powder drink. To accompany your protein, think greens! Yes, greens for breakfast to boost your vitamins, minerals and phyto-nutrients. Here's a great breakfast idea that's ready in minutes: Scrambled Eggs with spinach and tomatoes. Sauté a couple of tomatoes in olive oil, then add a large handful of spinach leaves and two beaten eggs and stir briefly to cook. Throw in a few herbs and a sprinkle pepper to taste and, hey presto! You have a quick, easy and nutritious breakfast.

How you begin will always have a bearing on where you end up. However if you are not fit and healthy now, you can change the path that has bought you thus far and leave behind a legacy of great self -change for others to be inspired by. It only takes two to three weeks to change your taste buds, but it may take you years to fend off cancer, or heart disease or lose those excess kilos. Change is merely a journey between where you are now and where you want to be. There is nothing to fear and everything to gain. The journey is the exciting adventure and just as important as the end.

Whatever your start in life, you can choose to be healthy now, and you have the knowledge the years before have given you....like your own encyclopaedia of you! So you are setting off on your journey well informed!

Although we cannot go back and start our lives from the beginning, (as much as we would like to with the benefit of hindsight) we can choose to make this a new beginning and start from now. Every seven years or so, we become essentially new people, because in that time, every cell in our body has been replaced by a new cell. Some cells are replaced in days, weeks or months so parts of us are regenerated nearly every day. This means we get rid of the old, as we do when we clear out our wardrobes, and we can learn to treat the new to a fabulous way of special care and attention. We have the choice to change how we are. All we have to do is step up and take hold of the reins...

Take Responsibility

"The price of greatness is responsibility."
— Winston Churchill

Because of the work I do, when I am socialising the conversation often turns to food, or issues regarding health. I rarely instigate such a conversation, after all I am officially off duty when socialising, but it gives me an idea of what it must be like to be a doctor at a dinner party! I listen to people go on and on about their lack of sleep, their aching joints, their problems with their husband/wife , the extra kilos they want to shed and even how ugly their fungal nail infection is on their toes, which is particularly tasteful over dinner! They moan away, sometimes for hours (I am a great listener), but I have a superb way to stop them in their tracks when I have had enough. I simply ask 'What are you going to do about it?' The sweet sound of silence is always swift to follow, coupled with a look of complete shock. 'What does she mean, what am I going to do about it?

Before you can change anything you are unhappy about in your life, you need to step up and take responsibility for where you are now. That is something people rarely realise and when it comes to health they are constantly complaining about it, looking for someone else to right it or some magic pill to fix it. Then they blame absolutely everything they can, when they are still not well.

Take a long hard look in the mirror. Your reflection is a true picture of all the life choices you have made up until now. Yes, I know that is harsh, but it is true. What you see staring back at you is a combination of your lifestyle choices. So what is it you do not like to see in the mirror? Perhaps your skin is not clear, or your eyes are bloodshot; maybe you have a spare tyre or two around your middle, or your hair is limp or thinning. Maybe your nails are broken or your stomach is bloated, your teeth are in poor condition or your backside has dropped! Maybe you look a lot older than how you would like to look, and/ or tired or unhappy. Be honest when you look at yourself. Don't be a critic, be a realist. Don't look at what you were born with, but what you have grown into.

Classic client examples: Mr Snuffleupagus who spoke to me about his diabetes which was reaching a point where dire implications were imminent. He said to me 'I know I drink a lot of beer, but it is not the beer that is the problem, it is the sugar. There is nothing I can do about this. Do you think you can help me?' Or Virginia Virginia who wanted to lose weight but did not want to give up her daily afternoon slice of cake, or her morning biscuits with her tea. She wanted to know what pills she could take to make her slim. Both were failing to take responsibility for where they were and they wanted someone or something else to fix their problems.

The easiest thing to do is to blame others for your present state, but do your best not to as this will not help you to do something about it. We have become a blame society, with the politicians out there leading the way, blaming everyone but themselves for the mess they have created. We blame the weather, money, the banks, the press, our partners, friends, parents, the car, the kids, our work, lack of time, even the poor dog gets the blame! We have forgotten how to take responsibility and admit that actually the problems we are experiencing might just be down to us!

> I, who will be known from here on in, as Big Bird, blamed all kinds of people and things for the state of my health when I was very ill 12 years ago. They had an effect, of course, as Big Bird had unwittingly, allowed them to. The doctors, the health system, the blood tests, my wretched ex-husband (polite version), my career, my finances, being a single mum, the banks, the courts, my best friend, my new partner......... they were all to blame. Then at the end of the day, when I learnt to stop blaming and take the control and responsibility I was able to stop wallowing in self-pity like a pathetic victim, and triumph in my ability to heal myself and my life. Now Big Bird couldn't be stronger, and all those things and people I use to blame, I now thank them for their valuable lessons which have lead me to my success. Big Bird flying high!

If you continue to blame others for the state of your health, you will be waiting for them to fix it too. Ahhhh my friend, here is one thing I have certainly learnt and that is that no one else will have quite the same interest in the way you feel as you. And others will certainly not have the enthusiasm to fix you either. Another person can't feel your pain, your discomfort, your stress, your hormones, your bloated stomach, your poor vision, your lack of energy, your difficulty concentrating, your lack of libido, your stuffy nose, your itchy skin, your anxiety, your depression or your lack of enjoyment in life. Only you can experience your feelings, so it needs to be you who does the deed and sorts it all out. Other people have their own problems and no matter how sympathetic they may appear to your cause, your issues are not their concern.

Maybe now is as good a time as any to take the responsibility for the state of your health. You can't continue to blame your limited time, lack of energy, kids, husband or Great Aunt Mary as it is down to you, my friend. Whether you are comfortable with this or not, wherever you are now it has all been your own doing. But, hey, let's not forget to always look on the bright side of life - this is marvellous news, because it means that as you have made all this, you have the power to change it all too! All you need to do is take the responsibility.

Of course taking responsibility does not mean fixing your health by yourself. It means picking up the reins and taking some action. Ask for help - doing this is a sign of strength, not a weakness. Start to read, research, go see your doctor, see a chiropractor, a nutritionist, a counsellor, your boss, talk to your family, take a walk, buy a healthy cook book, plant some vegetables, join AA, go to the dentist (eeeeek). If you are initially unsuccessful at getting the answers you need, keep searching and certainly do not give up at the first hurdle. Taking responsibility means that you yourself are taking positive action, to help you to live a wonderful life.

From today understand that you have control over your choices in life. Understand then, that you are the one responsible and face up to the responsibility. There is something quite revolutionary in doing this. You will feel empowered my friend. Once you feel like you have control, (which you do), no matter what you have been going through, or whatever your problem is, it will not seem anything like the tyrant it was before. Mind you, do not expect to have control over things that are out of your hands, for example - other people's lives, the weather, and the stock market or when your mother in law will choose to invade your home! Focus your energy on what you can control - your life - and make your life happen the way you want it to.

Before you go into full assault mode-this is not a time to be self-critical, but a time to ask questions. It is a time to treat yourself to a little TLC (tender loving care). It's unfair to beat yourself up, or feel upset with yourself for your situation. You are your best friend and we don't tend to beat up or upset best friends — least I hope you don't. Best friends need a bit of peace, love and understanding, (sounds like a song to me), so give a little of each to yourself.

The next time you visit the supermarket take a big breath and remember you are responsible for the food you choose to place in your trolley. A pack of chocolate digestives will not throw itself into your trolley and hold you at gun point to buy it. And I am pretty sure that processed ready meals don't leap out of the freezer and dive bomb into your trolley uninvited either. You can steer your trolley, even if the castors are really dodgy, away from the crisps, cakes and ready meals, and towards the fresh vegetables, fruit, meat, fish, nuts and seeds. Pick up some free range eggs, a little asparagus to steam, and some delicious dark chocolate to satisfy a sweet craving.

Did I say chocolate? Big Bird, really!! Well, apart from the fact that I am a woman, I am a self-confessed chocoholic, without shame! I am always happy to point out the amazing health benefits of a few squares of dark, cocoa rich chocolate! It is a plant....so it must be good for you, right? Yes, is the answer providing it is high in cocoa content...around 75% and that you do not eat too much of it to cancel out the health benefits as it does contain sugar and fat- unless you eat the really raw stuff. But still on a positive note. It is mood enhancing, high in protein, high in antioxidants, rich in vitamins A, B1, B2, B3, C, E and pantothenic acid, sulphur, and magnesium. It promotes heart health, circulation and focus. It is also an aphrodisiac....well it is easy to love, let's put it that way! Eat a couple of squares every day if you want and feel no guilt. Melt a couple of squares and dip chunks of fruit in for a delicious sweet treat. Now where did I put that bar....?

The next time you are faced with a stressful situation, it is your choice whether you act or react (see my chapter on Stress). The next time coffee with a certain friend leaves you feeling drained and miserable, remember you have the choice to say no if she asks to bend your ear again...albeit over coffee. Tomorrow when you wake up, you have the choice to greet your day with a smile and do your best to put a positive spin on it, or be your normal grumpy self, and moan about everything in sight. When you get out of bed feeling as tired as you went in, you can continue in this way or seek another way to feel full of energy, rested and raring to go. You can choose to take the stairs rather than the lift and you can walk to the local shop, rather than jumping into your car, if you choose to. When you are faced with the question 'What is for dinner tonight?' You could pick up the phone and order another take out, or you could muster up something quick and healthy. As a responsible adult, you decide where your life will take you and how the journey will be. Your life is your responsibility, it makes perfect sense to choose to make the very best of it........

Don't worry, be happy!

"Happiness depends upon ourselves."
— Aristotle

Let's begin this section about happiness by getting one thing straight my friend - it's always good to set the rules of play before you begin wouldn't you agree? - Happiness is not a commodity that you can buy from a supermarket or order from the internet, or pop in to buy from the late night garage, although people speak about it as if it is something we can 'get'. Mind you, wouldn't that be great, to do the weekly shop and buy a little happiness along with the mobile phone top up and lottery ticket? Perhaps if you could purchase some happiness there would be no need to spend your money on a lottery ticket!

However we all know the saying, 'money can't buy happiness' and this is true because it is a feeling. You can't purchase it, no one can give it to you and no one can take it from you, despite what you may have been lead to believe. Happiness is your feeling. It belongs to you. Of course surroundings and people can have an impact on your feelings, but you are the one who 'allows' any impact to occur.

Your outer world is merely a reflection of your inner state my friend, which is great if you know and understand that you can change it. It has taken me many years to understand this reality, but now that I have (finally!) grasped it, my feelings of happiness far surpass anything I have ever known. I spent many years feeling unhappy and blaming circumstances and those around me for 'making' me unhappy. Of course they did not 'make' me unhappy, however cruel they seemingly were. I chose to allow feelings of unhappiness to engulf my soul. I did not understand that I was the one with the power to make myself feel miserable and unhappy. I also did not understand that I was the one with the ultimate power to change things!

This means that happiness is solely down to you. Easy for me to say and you are right, it is easy for me to say....in reality it is not so easy to grasp. However, she hastily adds, like anything in life, things are as easy or as difficult as you choose to make them.

The challenges of this world are sent to us all, no matter what title we hold, how rich or poor we are, what job we do, or, how many children we have or don't have. Every day challenges are sent our way. If you embrace every challenge, and rise to the challenge, you will prove yourself a winner every time – even if it takes a while to get there! Be glad of the challenges because you will learn something new each time and the day you stop learning is the day your life is over, so be content to be a good student my friend!

Some people (I was one), see these challenges as difficulties which, by the very word, makes life feel a miserable struggle. If you replace the word difficult with challenge it changes the whole concept and we can all rise to a challenge!

My friend, there is a body and mind connection which all the experts talk about. Of course you realised that your body and mind are connected being as your head is attached to your body, didn't you?! But just in case you didn't realise that the two were connected, it is a fact that your mind can have an effect on your body and your body can have an effect on your mind. The things we focus on, and whatever we think about inevitably becomes our reality and affects the entire way we feel and, as a result, can have an impact on our health – for better or worse. Just like when we are in pain, or are suffering from a sickness, it can make us feel down in the dumps. And when we are feeling extremely happy we feel like we can run and jump and conquer anything all day.

To demonstrate this point try this little exercise : Sit up straight, smile, lift up your head so your eyes are higher than the horizon, push your shoulders back, breath steadily and deeply, and think about a time or an event that made you feel happy. Concentrate on this stance and these feelings for a few minutes. I am sure you will immediately begin to feel much better than you did before you started. You may even find an ache or a pain in your body seems to ease a little. If you now reverse all that, lose the smile, put your head down, hunch your shoulders and think about something that makes you feel miserable, you may even start to feel sick. This is the movie star trick to crying or laughing on screen. They learn to put their self in a particular state, and you too have the power to do this and you use it many times unwittingly! Think about how you could change things if you used this in a beneficial way every day!

Did you know there are more nerve connections from your brain to your digestive system than there are to any other part of your body? Well now you know and it may explain why you get a dodgy belly when you feel threatened by an external stimulus, or those butterflies in your stomach when you are nervously excited; or those pangs of hunger when you think you will have to go without food – the diet syndrome! Your digestive system is the engine of your body. It is where your immune system has its base and where your health truly begins and ends due to the very fact that you need a healthy immune system to have a healthy body. A disrupted digestive system, such as constant indigestion, bloating, pain, acid reflux, constipation or diarrhoea, will have an immediate effect on your immunity and hence your health and so often this can be influenced heavily by the state of your emotional health. People who are generally happy tend to have less digestive upsets and thus healthier immune systems. Being happy is essential for good health and, of course, it goes without saying that it is a great way to be!

Once again the words are wise, but how exactly do you change your levels of happiness? How do you make that transformation from a place where so much in life makes you feel miserable, to a place in life where you are content, at peace and full of incredibly happy feelings? It all starts, like everything and anything, by making a decision to change and taking action. However, it does not necessarily mean struggling to change how you feel by yourself. If you are suffering from depression or anxiety, for instance, you need to seek professional help from those who are trained to help you. If you feel you are stuck in a rut, perhaps consulting with a Life Coach will help you forward, or perhaps you need to consult with a financial expert if you have financial problems. If you are unhappy because you are overweight perhaps a personal trainer or a nutritionist would be useful to give you advice about diet and exercise. What is down to you is to take the decision to do something about the way you feel and seek the help you need (no one can help you if they do not know you need it).

The Telly Monster took that decision one day and requested a Skype consultation with me to talk about all that was bothering him and to share with me how miserable he was feeling. He had been suffering for many years with ME, a condition where you have long term chronic fatigue, muscular pain, joint pain and disturbed sleep patterns. He was unable to work, lived alone and felt lonely and isolated. He was very unhappy. Of course, it is understandable to be unhappy when life is seemingly so bleak, but there is always a light at the end of every tunnel. The first thing we worked on was acceptance of where the Telly Monster was in his life. Once he had learnt to accept his illness, rather than kicking against it, we were able to look at the internal stories he was feeding himself every day - stories about how his life was a failure and how he would never be happy. The Telly Monster began to feed himself different stories, stories about how he had been on a journey of self-discovery , how he had the power to re -create his life with a new look and how he could achieve things every day, even if they were small. Together we worked on his diet and he began a programme of supplementation which helped his physical and mental state to improve. The Telly Monster began to realise, as he got stronger, that everything was within his control, even the ME and that he could be the author of his life and create the happiness he was seeking. He took up a light exercise program, taught himself new skills on the computer and joined a local networking group to create a social network that would also bring him business. Now he is heard to quote my words to others about how wonderful life is. He has a successful computer based business which he works from the comfort of his own home, so that it fits in with his energy levels. He works alongside his ME which is improving still, and accepts he has to pace himself in order to make the most of every day – like we all should! The Telly Monster now shares his home with the love of his life which is the icing on the cake. One happy Telly Monster!

Do not expect miracles my friend, or life to instantly be different when you make a conscious decision to change things. Rome was not built in a day, but it was worth the continual effort! It will take you a while to be in the 'happy' zone, and it is all about the journey in between.

I had a mental and physical breakdown when I was sick all those years ago, and it took poor Big Bird some months to bounce back, and some years to truly kick the negative feelings. Even now I still have the odd days where I prefer to be a hermit and not to see anyone, or speak to anyone and I still have my days where the thought of going to buy a bottle of water from the supermarket fills me with dread. Unfounded fears, and Big Bird knows it, but it is still there, albeit very much in the background and not enough to interfere and have a negative effect on life – no chance! I accept I have been left with this slight weakness, and by accepting it I do not beat myself up for it! I merely allow myself to be as I feel, and do my best to live my day alongside it, not against it. It works well!

I was explaining about my breakdown to Zoe who was suffering from acute anxiety as she felt she was very much alone in her fight. After Zoe listened, almost in disbelief that I had been through such an experience, she asked me how I had managed to change how I was feeling. To be perfectly honest, I did not have professional help, I did not take medication, but a doctor I saw told me I had the power to overcome what I was going through. That was it. So I decided (I made a decision), after a few days of thinking of the doctor's simple statement (stemming from what I initially thought was a huge lack of understanding), that he was right and I took each day slowly and worked on finding the solutions to my problems. I managed my initial change really well and, even though I still had physical health issues to deal with, my mental state improved significantly. The real pivotal point of change came a few years later when I studied Life Coaching, Cognitive Behavioural Therapy and Neuro Linguistic Programming. So, although I did not have professional help as such, by learning I was given all the pointers necessary for me to finish what I had started alone. I must say, I did a great job!

So it all starts with a decision to change and seeking the tools you need to do the job. It's a bit like that DIY job you have been putting off for so long. Once you decide to begin and have the right tools to hand you will be on a roll (and the other half will be off your back!). Being happy is an internal state and that's the bit you need to work on. Don't believe that the bigger house, the Mercedes, the new boyfriend or the holiday, which are all wonderful of course, will 'make' you happy. Your inner state is your true happiness. Learning to make small changes in the way you feel, the way you act and the way you think can make a huge difference. Of course, there is no reason to give up on the Mercedes, or the boyfriend!

A little word if I may about something that is essential for you to know and understand. Life is full of balance. The world has balance. Just look around and you will see the sun and the rain, the hot and the cold, life and death, sickness and health, gluttony and starvation, wealth and poverty etc. It is the same in everyone's life. There is good and bad, happiness and sadness, laughter and tears, love and hate, riches and not a penny in the bank! And so on. So you need to know and accept that you will have balance of everything in your life too, including some sadness along with the happiness, which is perfectly natural and normal – it is the way of the world!

Being grateful for what you have is one of the cornerstones for emotional happiness. Look around you and learn to see the things to be grateful for. Sure you may be broke and in a job you do not like, but perhaps you have a loving family, good friends at work, and flowers in your garden, plus a body that functions pretty well. Spending time focusing on what is not right will only enhance its powers over you. Focusing on what is right, and feeling gratitude for these things however, will help bring feelings of peace, which in turn will help you feel happier.

Having a positive outlook will certainly go a long way with feelings of happiness and will assist a fit and healthy body and mind. There is plenty of research out there to prove that it works. Being positive about life will keep your mind healthier and in so doing, your body. Of course, we cannot be positive all the time, but making a consistent effort to be more positive about life in general will certainly pay dividends.

Beans and lentils combine protein and starchy carbohydrates which gives them a very low GI and helps keep energy levels stable. They are an excellent source of B vitamins which are important vitamins to boost a positive state. Instead of using meat, make chilli con carne with kidney beans and chickpeas, or try a bolognaise made with lentils and served on brown rice (another great source of B vitamins).

When we repeat over and over a statement to our self, our body responds to it as it creates a neural pathway. So if you keep telling yourself that you are fat, for instance, the body will respond and you will be or remain fat, no matter how hard you work at that diet! Changing neural pathways takes effort because it is like retraining your brain, but it can be done. Feed your mind with the statements you want to be true in your life, like 'I am fit and healthy'. Repeat it over and over again and do your best to not let the more negative statements take centre stage. It is like learning a new language, so practice makes perfect my friend.

Take time to relax, meditate, and be kind to yourself. Being kind to yourself - and to others of course - will elevate the feelings of happiness. Being kind is good for your heart and your soul! Meditation reduces stress and anxiety, plus it improves your quality of life and boosts your immune system. Meditation has been shown to decrease anger and improve sleep and it gives you time to breathe. I mean, seriously, at what point in your day do you stop just to breath?

If there is one prescription that should be handed out by all doctors, alternative and conventional, it is a prescription for people to smile. Smiling not only helps you to feel happy, which in turn has a positive effect on your health, but it makes you look younger and healthier too! A smile is extremely contagious my friend. Try it and you will see. Smile at someone today and see if they don't smile back. Just that simple act will lift your spirits and you will lift someone else's too. Smiling exercises the facial muscles, helping to keep them toned, which, if you think about it, should be part of your natural beauty regime. And whilst you are smiling, how about laughing too? Laughter is a common remedy for all ailments, and you should always leave some room for laughter in your daily life. Not only will you feel better, but, they say, you will also live longer and I will go along with that.

"There's nothing like deep breaths after laughing that hard. Nothing in the world like a sore stomach for the right reasons."
— Stephen Chbosky

Choose to be in environments and around people that increase your probability of happiness. Definitely do your best to stay away from the people who increase your feelings of unhappiness, I mean, why would you want to be around such people? I understand that this can be difficult if you are at work and it is your colleague or boss that brings you feelings of total misery. If this is the case then you need to find a way to lighten the situation – for instance, (I and many of my clients love this strategy), in your mind use your imagination to turn the tyrant into a cartoon character complete with voice to match - it certainly lightens what is causing you angst. Perhaps you could find a way to move to another department, or, in time, change where you work. If it is a friend who brings unhappiness, or even someone closer to home, find a way to be out of their company rather than in it. Do your best to socialise with the people who make you feel good about yourself and who help you to laugh and see the brighter side of life!

When I was twenty seven years old I was raped in my own home. My eldest son, who was six at the time, was asleep upstairs Not a very pleasant thing for Big Bird to have to endure or to live with after. I carried it for years. That, and some other daunting events, not all them dissimilar. However, the day I decided to forgive these people, was the day I started to truly live again. The feeling of lightness is incredible and today I hold no ill feeling towards them. I have never condoned their acts, nor will I ever do so, but by forgiving them I released myself from my own torture and am able to love life again to the full!

Learn to forgive others. Holding onto anger, resentment or feelings of wrong doing by others doesn't really do anything beneficial for you. It serves no great purpose, but it can be very destructive to your physical and mental health. We all make mistakes, or do things that are not considered 'right' by another individual, but we have all asked for forgiveness too. Forgiving others releases you. It does not condone what they have done, but it does lift a weight from your shoulders. Even if you do not forgive someone to their face, forgive them in your mind, or write down your forgiveness and then let the feeling go. You will feel happier after!

Spread the lurv man! Love will enhance your happiness. You know how it feels when you go somewhere you love, or when you are in the arms of someone you love, or you are eating something you love! You feel happy. Do your best to love as much as you can and as many things around you as you can. Be a total lurv bug and most of all, love yourself.....

Love yourself.....exactly the way you are

"Love yourself - accept yourself - forgive yourself - and be good to yourself, because without you the rest of us are without a source of many wonderful things."
— Leo F. Buscaglia

Because you're gorgeous, because you're worth it, because you are the person you are. Love yourself my friend, every last bit of you, from the top of your head to the tips of your toes and all those cracking, wobbly bits in between. It is all yours, and all yours to love, accept and respect. You were born a wonderful human being, and you still are, even if you have grown fatter, skinnier, taller or shorter than you would like to be. Love is good for your health, and loving you will bring so many healthy dividends.

Regardless of anything you do, and what you look like my friend, it's all about recognising your inherent worth and creating a life that does you justice. First you need to accept exactly who you are. Acceptance will bring you peace and put pay to any internal wars you have going on. I acknowledge that this can be a bit of a challenge at the best of times, and on a bad day, when things have not been going your way, your self-acceptance can be truly challenged. But as we always look on the bright side of life, we can all nurture some pretty decent self- acceptance if we put our mind to it and see it as a skill we can practice and improve. A great way to start is to accept that we are not one hundred percent perfect. (Sorry if that came as a shock!) But then who is? It can be a relief when we accept this!

> When a client comes to me with an illness, be it IBS, a problem with allergies, cancer, multiple sclerosis or Parkinson's disease, the first thing I ask them to do, providing the diagnosis has been confirmed by tests of course, is to accept what they have. No one can deal reasonably with anything unless there is a level of acceptance. Once acceptance has been reached, inner peace follows, which makes for a stronger foundation on which to heal and sort out the issue.

We all need to accept that sometimes we may do things that aren't really what we would want to do and that things may not always be what we would want them to be. We may mess up! We should accept that we make mistakes and that sometimes we behave in a way that, with after- thought, we may not necessarily like. We have all been there I presume? (Hoping that it is not only me!) There may be a part or two of our bodies that we would not consider perfect (or not to our liking) and sometimes our body does not always respond in the way we would wish. But as we accept where we are in life, even if we have a serious illness or an addiction, then we can let go of the past and the things we cannot control. When we are able to do this we find ourselves in the driving seat, able to take action to make changes and we can focus our energy on that which we can control which is all empowering my friend!

Accept who you are, exactly as you are and once you do, you can fall in love with yourself. Learning to love yourself is great. Being in love with yourself is even greater! Make it the greatest romance of your life. Tattoo a love heart on your brain with your name in the very centre of it. When you love and accept yourself, you will find others are likely to accept and love you too. But if they don't it doesn't really matter as that is a matter for them! What matters is for you to continue loving and accepting who you are. Loving yourself will open up a whole new world.

By the way, mistakes are not as bad as they are made out to be. Mistakes give us something to learn from, grow from and heal from- which is all good my friend!

Our imperfections my friend, are as wonderful as our perfections. They make us unique. Furthermore, what one person would view as an imperfection, another would see as perfection. Have you ever wondered what a handsome man you know has seen in the ugly woman he is dating? Or vice versa? We each see a different perspective of the same image and so our views are different .Did you realise for all that time you spend running yourself down in front of the mirror, that if someone else had your 'assets' perhaps they would be praising them?

Be as kind to yourself as you would be to the love of your life and your best friend. As you will read more than once in this book, you are your best friend. You began your life with you and you will end it with you. You are the only person who will be with you throughout the entire journey of your life. Through your ups, your downs, your successes, your embarrassing moments, your marriages, your birthdays, your happy and sad times, your breakfast, lunch and supper times, your moments of glory and your times of defeat. This is a relationship that is truly valid both in sickness and in health. Wow, what a best friend to share all that with you! To love and to cherish as this is a person whose wonderful tolerance and unrivalled staying power with you is beyond what any other person could possibly ever offer. Recognise this. Don't be mean to that lovely friend, instead find gratitude inside and give as much love as you can. The love is well and truly earned over and over again – above and beyond any call of duty! It is time to celebrate exactly who you are! Pop the champagne cork my friend and have a party in your honour! (Any excuse, me!)

Being as you are one heck of a hero (even if you have only just realised it!) it seems a shame to spend too much time criticizing yourself. You always do the best you can, and that is all that can ever be asked of you. Throw out the inner critic (I am sure you have one in your head who is never tired or on holiday) and let in the admirer. If you believe your inner critic is always speaking the truth, it is time to allow in some doubt! Next time your critic tells you that you are not good enough, throw back an answer of 'You want to bet?' When you find yourself staring in the mirror having a go at your nose, or your hips, or your lack of biceps, smile back at the image and do an admiring twirl and tell yourself how gorgeous you are instead. Praise your body for carrying you around all day, thank it for its efforts, its care, and its tireless loyalty to yourself and tell it that you love it. Quieten down the critic, allow its voice to become a whisper, and let the admirer speak up with confidence.

I presume you know what I mean by an inner critic? I am sure you do. It's that chirpy little voice that pipes up in your head and keeps telling you that you are fat, or that you are stupid, or that you don't have any talent, or you could not possibly do that because you are just not up to it! This ever so annoying voice belongs to your Critical Little Devil. Just where does he get all this rubbish from? He has written a book over the years that contains your self- limiting beliefs. Beliefs that you have listened to about yourself, picked up from your parents, your peers, your teachers, the world in general and, bless that Critical Little Devil, he has learnt them all! What a pain this voice can be. If you are not careful it will hold you back from achieving and being all you have ever dreamed of. Criticise, criticise, criticise. That's all it does. Bla bla bla. And it's not like you have not been listening or that he says anything new is it? But do you know the worst thing? It's the fact that you have chosen to listen to him! Oh yes you have!!!

Time to realise that enough is enough and remove this little devil, wouldn't you agree my friend? Let's use our imagination...... Imagine two little cartoon figures sitting on each of your shoulders, you've seen them before I am sure in the likes of 'Tom and Jerry' cartoons. Neatly perched and feeling rather confident on your right shoulder is your Critical Little Devil. He is sitting there on a fluffy red rug, legs crossed, ever so smug, with his pitch fork in his hand (which is ready to poke you in your ribs each time he criticises to really drive the message home). Look at him, he just thinks he is so cool. Oh watch him now as he practices his break dancing! He is really super comfortable where he is, but, secret, we are about to shove him out of his comfort zone. Oh yes, exciting isn't it when you know the plot??!.

So if your Critical Little Devil is sitting on your right shoulder, then tell me my friend, who do you think sits on your left shoulder? Your Guardian Angel? Sorry wrong answer but it's a very easy mistake to make! It's not a Guardian Angel, as such, although it will take good care of you. It's a powerful mini version of you! It's so power packed, it is as if all the power has been vacuum packed inside a mini you! What is more you are looking absolutely fabulous my friend! Love the outfit and your hair....have you just had it re styled? It really suits you like that!

All will be going just great until a situation arises which will give your Critical Little Devil a perfect platform to open his mouth and throw obscenities at you. The pitch fork is ready to jab you in your ribs, but sadly for the Critical Little Devil, he hasn't seen mini you saunter up behind. I use the term saunter because you know exactly how great and powerful you are and you don't want to run and mess up your fab new hair- do! Before the Critical Little Devil can get the first word out, you pull the fluffy rug from under his feet and watch him tumble all the way down to the floor. Just when he thinks things can't get any worse, mini you notices he had dropped his pitch fork before he fell, so you toss it over board and it lands directly on his head, leaving him with a host of little birds flying in circles above him. Ah ha! You are the all- time powerful, all time fabulous, all time capable, talented, and totally in control person. (Victory lap of both shoulders beautifully performed and your hair still looks perfect!)

But don't be lured into a false sense of security quite yet my friend. Like any little villain, your Critical Little Devil doesn't give up the ghost quite that easily and will find his way back up to his comfort zone. However, each time he does this you will be ready and you will just find different ways of knocking him off his perch, until eventually, he will begin to lose his power and take the right decision to give up. Then you will stand there smug, in control, responsible for yourself, and feeling powerful and unstoppable. Yes! (Accompanied by a winning punch into the air!)

But I hear you cry, if I stop all the criticism, accept myself as I am and tell myself that I love myself, that means I have to be happy with me as I am, and I am not. Acceptance is not resignation my friend, so let me help you on that one. Do you remember your first car? Do you remember how much you loved it, cared for it, polished it and was proud of it? I am sure it was your pride and joy! I certainly remember mine, a good solid, heavy beast of a car, cream in colour, no spoilers, no rear seatbelts, or electric windows, no power steering, in fact it was like driving a tank. Awww….. My lovely Austin Maxi, my Henrietta! I was in love with her. But it did not stop me upgrading her when the time was right. I am sure you have also upgraded your car, your house, your mobile phone, your first boyfriend etc. Loving yourself as you are does not mean you have to remain exactly as you are. If that were the case what would be the point of education and evolution? Maybe it is time to upgrade yourself, but if you don't love and appreciate what you already have, why would this world give you the opportunity to have something more?

Here is a little scenario to help you understand the point I am trying my best to make. Imagine the time you present your child with a new bike that you have spent several months planning and paying for, but instead of the bike being met with joy, your child is disappointed and critical of the model you have chosen. When you see the disappointment and the lack of gratitude, your first thought would probably be 'ungrateful child.' And as he asks for something better, with a loader bell, and bigger wheels, you will probably tell him to like what he has and be thankful for it. However, as time passes and you see him taking time to make it sparkle every Sunday and racing it everywhere he can, you would probably be tempted to buy him a loader bell, or may even plan to buy the model he really wants for his next birthday. But on the other hand, if you saw the bike left to rust in the back yard, never ridden, and neglected, I am sure that you would have little enthusiasm to upgrade the model in any way shape or form. Whatever is not appreciated will depreciate. The same goes for yourself. Love and appreciate what you have now and maybe by doing this, opportunities will come your way to upgrade the parts you feel you need to.

I had a client, Oscar the Grouch, who hated himself in many ways. Oscar was a very angry person, which affected every aspect of his daily waking hours and also those hours when he was meant to sleep! On reflection, his life was a mixture of complex matters of the heart, a poor financial position, general ill health and chaotic business. We didn't work at all on Oscar's health for a few weeks, just on self-love. When he finally accepted he needed to love himself, and started to practise the very same, everything around him moved in a positive direction. We had to start small, for example, with Oscar the Grouch accepting that he had beautiful eyes. However we built on this until he saw himself in a completely different light. Oscar's whole persona changed as he learnt to love himself and the calm in his life that followed was really quite remarkable. I have to say, if Oscar the Grouch could do this, then so can you. Step, by step, slowly, slowly. Dear Oscar learnt to stop hating, which is a negative, destructive emotion and force, and began to love.

You can alter the perceptions you have about yourself if you choose to and then perhaps your path forward will also be altered. You are a magnificent human being, unique like your DNA, blessed in many ways, and you should honour yourself. Understand that your body works for you, it is your best friend, not your enemy and give it the love it deserves, after all without it, where would you be? You have some amazing strengths that have got you this far, concentrate your mind on these.

If you have a healthy respect, appreciate your best friend, and love it with all your heart, you can begin to make changes my friend. If you have spent your life criticising yourself, it is going to take you a little time to undo this learnt behaviour and turn it around. Please try not to expect miracles to happen. Loving takes time, so give yourself plenty of time.

Patience and understanding is required, as is perseverance, hope, belief, desire and enthusiasm. Accept the progress you make, whatever the pace and don't rush to become something too quickly. The slow and the steady are the ones that always win the race.....even though this is not a race!

It all starts with a conscious decision to love yourself and this needs a good bit of positive reinforcement every which way you can. Begin small and simple, by telling yourself every morning and every evening that you love, appreciate and respect yourself. Make this your twice daily affirmation – the minute you wake up and directly before you go to sleep. It will set you up for the day ahead and give thought for your sub conscious whilst you are asleep.

Affirmations are incredibly powerful and are a great way to retrain the way you think. An affirmation is a positive statement, set in the present tense, such as' I am happy and content with my life.' Affirmations make you conscious of your thoughts. To affirm means to say something positively. It means to declare firmly and assert something to be true. Affirmations are statements where you assert that what you want to be true is true. When you repeat such a statement over and over again, eventually your brain will begin to believe it and act upon it. Affirmations can be used for anything in life and my clients use them to regain health, lose weight, and change their lives in general. I am not aware of anyone for whom affirmations have not made a difference. I, myself, affirm my life, especially when I need to bring about more certainty in an area.

Shall I waffle here and tell you a little story of how

affirmations worked for Big Bird? Yes why not. I lived in Crete for seven years and then moved back to the UK due to family reasons. I was not at home any longer in the UK, the weather, the system, the food, life in general and I struggled to come to terms with life there. My soul belonged in Crete, it was where I felt at home and I began to battle with myself and life in the UK, which left me feeling miserable, defeated, lost and uncomfortable. I believed I would never be able to see my beautiful Crete again, that it was impossible to find my way back there, to live the life I felt I was born to live .The more I believed I was destined to live in the UK under the grey skies, the more my life was set to continue in that way. One huge blessing about residing in the UK was the time I had to study – a gift I will be forever thankful for, and like I said, I studied Life Coaching and NLP which convinced me to a) change my attitude towards the UK, and b) start to affirm the changes I wanted to see in my life. I learnt acceptance of where my life had bought me, gratitude for what I had and the knowledge of affirmations that would change my life.

I began to affirm that I would be back in Crete for a holiday within less than a year. I made it a goal and affirmed it every day. I affirmed I would have the money to make this happen, and the strength to hold my dream true. Sure enough within eight months I was back in Crete for a glorious week. Magic, whether it be hippy, weird or not! I then set myself to task on affirming a future on my island, a way to combine my family in the UK and my life where I belonged. For the next couple of years I visited Crete nine times! I began to make a name for the work I did and advertised my time on the island to grow a client base. Then one day an opportunity presented itself which would take me to the island for a year, whilst going back to the UK every couple of months to spend family time….. and here we are! I can't divulge the next part of my life or I will have to kill you, but rest assured, the affirmations are in place and I am working on my future, slowly bringing it to pass.

Waffle over, let's get back to loving you! Loving yourself is very much about having self -respect. A simple way to get this underway is to take time and care to dress and groom your body every day. Dressing well, whatever fashion that is for you, will in itself give you greater confidence and make you feel a whole lot better in your health too. If you dress in clothes that make you feel uncomfortable or worthless, your health, body and mind, will feel the same, but if you dress yourself in clothes that make you feel good, you will feel great. Remember the body mind connection thingy the experts, including me, bang on about - Feel good in your mind and you will feel good in your body. Look good in your body and you will feel fabulous in your mind. Your appearance is a reflection to the outside world of how much you care and value yourself. Value yourself above all others and show it off with a sense of purpose to the outside world.

Before your morning shower take five deep breathes and then do a few stretches. Have a quick, vigorous body brush (this is as good for you guys as it is you girls) to remove dead skin and improve circulation. Skin brushing is exercise for the skin and brushing removes the top layer which helps to eliminate uric acid crystals and various other acid materials from the body. By keeping the skin active you help it in its battle to rid the body of impurities. Continue to stimulate the skin by use a natural body scrub, such as olive oil and sugar to deep clean, remove impurities, and give yourself smooth, radiant skin. You will feel very zingy after and ready to take on the world. And you will feel even more zingy if you end with a few seconds of a cold water shower!!!

If you are a woman take the time to do your make up if you wear it, or if you don't, make sure you pay extra special care to your facial skin so you feel like you are glowing. Take care to pay attention to the feel of your skin, and caress it with love as you would a baby. A diet high in sugar causes premature aging. The skin looks dull, is no longer smooth, loses elasticity quickly and is more prone to inflammation (redness). Your fork is your best way to remain looking young and beautiful. Antioxidants help prevent sugar from attaching to protein so eat lots of antioxidant rich whole foods. These are vegetables and fruit that have rich colours for example: dark green, purple, red, blue, orange and yellow. Choose spinach, carrots, squash, sweet potatoes, red/yellow peppers, kale, mangoes, papayas, blueberries, raspberries, strawberries etc. Add to that eggs, legumes, salmon and tuna and you will be eating yourself young and beautiful – which you will love!

Get out in the fresh air and breathe deeply. Take a deep breath through your nose, and let it out easily through your mouth. Or, inhale and exhale through your nose, mentally counting "in-two-three, out-two-three," and then "pause-two-three." During the pause, don't breathe in or out; just rest comfortably. Take in the sights and sounds and indulge your senses. Walking is one of the best forms of exercise, and I am sure that you can fit a ten minute stroll into your day. Begin to reshape your body, strengthen your energy and clear your mind.

Forget comparing yourself to others! There is no comparison. They are they, you are you, it is that simple. Makes life a little less complicated doesn't it!? Every time you see another person you feel has something better to offer the world than you have, stop and think again. Do they really have something you don't? I doubt it very much. And believe me, what you think you see and know about another person, even your other best friend (first best friend being you, of course), behind closed doors is usually something very different – and they are probably wishing they were more like someone else, with someone else's life and someone else's car! Why is there always such an obsession to think that others around are so much more than ourselves? It makes greater sense to have the obsession with ourselves, spending as much time and focus on loving our own fabulous self.

Learn to let go of past events as this is now a new, fresh beginning for you. There are a lot of us who have had some pretty hard times to come through, but instead of using these times to hinder your way forward, choose to learn from the challenges and appreciate how you have grown and changed from them. Forgive others and most importantly, forgive yourself. You are only human!

Eat a diet that will aid your feelings of self -worth. Processed foods offer your brain no nutrients to help it see life in a positive form and it is much easier to be a miserable toad if you feed your brain junk. Plus of course, your health and weight will suffer, neither of which will serve to make you love yourself. Of course you could go to a deserted island where there is no junk food to hand, but that suggestion may be a little far -fetched, so how about a more feasible answer – simply eating foods that provide the nutrients your body needs for you to feel more positive. By filling up on nature's super foods you will soothe your body, lift your spirits and see off any naughty little cravings for good. What a way to show you how much you love you!

Packed with potassium which helps to balance the body's fluids and blood pressure, bananas are a great mood booster. Slice them up on your porridge, or oven bake for a great dessert served with natural yogurt and nuts (or a square or two of melted dark chocolate) – which also makes a tasty 'I love me' breakfast.

Self -care is very important and aids self- love. Some people are not so kind to themselves abusing their body with stress, late nights, eating poor food choices, no exercise or too much, continually putting others before their own needs, and a lack of interest in how they are .I am sure this is not you my friend? Although many people think it is, it is not selfish to look after yourself, but indeed a self- less act. You can't give what you do not have, so unless you love and care for yourself, you will not be able to give the same for others. Likewise, if you do not love and care for yourself, why would you expect others to love and care for you? The more you work on and invest in yourself, the more you will be able to give to this world, the more the world will give to you and that is one beautiful win, win situation!

Its action stations again my friend! Book a massage, take a long hot soak in a candle lit bathroom, sort out your wardrobe, have your hair cut, take some nutritional advice, spend some time with friends, join a dance class. Cut back your hours at work, re think how you run your day and take time to relax. Express yourself perhaps through writing a short story, or painting a picture. Be creative. Have something all about you to look forward to each day, however small it may be. Write a gratitude list for all the amazing things you have (you have so many things to be grateful for my friend) .Work as steadily as you can at loving you, exactly as you are.

Remember every morning during your very tedious journey to work, just how lucky you are, that despite all your short comings, someone loves you. And that someone is you. Focus your attention on saying something nice to yourself and decide what special thing you will do for yourself later in the day. Think of all the times you have taken yourself for granted and make up for it with a little tender loving care. Appreciate your life. Invest in yourself, accept who you are, love yourself, and you will become a beacon of light in this world.

Stress – The Silent Killer

"I promise you nothing is as chaotic as it seems. Nothing is worth diminishing your health. Nothing is worth poisoning yourself into stress, anxiety, and fear."
— Steve Maraboli

I cannot begin to tell you how much I love it when people tell me that they do not suffer from stress - it's almost as bizarre as when people tell me that I don't know what it is like to be under stress! Stress is an issue we can all relate to and are all subject to. However we can be - a) the victims of stress and as a result, maybe stress related disease, or we could- b) learn to manage stress so that it has minimal impact upon our being. Obviously I practise scenario b)- managing stress so that it has little impact, which, I am sure, is why people believe I do not know what stress is like. I must admit, I am pretty happy about the fact that I manage it so well now –it was not always this way. But, the real question is, what scenario is yours?

Stressful situations are all around us my friend. The moment you are born the stress of the big wide world flies out of the air towards you as you are slapped on your butt to get you to yell (well, breathe clearly actually).From then on it doesn't really stop, it's just a different style of slap each time and you yell in different ways in response. It is exactly the type of response that will determine how well you deal, or don't deal with stress. The less able you are at dealing with stress the bigger the impact it will have upon your health, mental and physical, and hence your life.

There is a good side to stress as well as a bad side..... just to be fair to stress. In small doses stress can be a good thing as it motivates you through your day and towards your goals. It can boost your memory, improve how your heart works, fortify the immune system and protect your body from infection. A quick surge of stress gives your body and brain a boost and can literally, starve off disease. It is like a roadside repair crew turning up! Stress increases your senses so that your focus is hugely enhanced, which could be life-saving, such as jumping out of the way of a moving car! Stress is key to survival, but in small doses. As with anything in life my friend, there is a need for balance. Too little stress and you are hanging around feeling bored and unmotivated. Too much stress and you are wired and tired and heading for a heart attack...or something similar!

We live in a stressful era, possibly the most stressful period humans have ever experienced, well so they say. When I look back through history I am pretty sure it was a wee bit stressful to live through the French Revolution or the First World War, and I believe that stress, like anything else, is relevant to the era we live in and the lifestyle we lead. However, stress is the greatest issue that modern humans have to deal with and one of the biggest causes of illness. This can be serious enough to lead to death – we just don't realise it. Stress costs industries and companies billions, causes relationships to break up, children to hate school and people to go AWOL from life! It's there all around us, but it does not need to have dire implications unless you allow it to. You can learn to manage stress and keep it in its proper place.

Prolonged bouts of severe stress have a negative impact on your health. Stress is implicated in every type of health issue from high blood pressure to infertility. Stress affects the body and mind in many ways, and everyone experiences stress differently. Not only can overwhelming stress lead to serious mental and physical health problems, it can also take a toll on your relationships at home, work, and school. I am sure that if your daily grind is full of stress then come the time for night time activities, sadly you would have more enthusiasm to clean the dishes than make passionate love to your partner. Stress, along with very large pants, tends to be a real passion killer!

Even though we can all relate to the term 'stress' , most of us do not really understand what it is. If your doctor was to tell you your ill health was caused by stress you would probably think he or she was lacking an interest in a proper diagnosis and brushing your problems aside. The reality is my friend, your doctor could well be right. The big issue is, how much damage has your stress already caused you? And can you limit the effects it has in the future?

First and foremost it is important for you to understand what stress does to your body so that you can begin to understand its effects, so let us delve gently into an explanation. When you encounter stress the adrenal glands, which sit neatly on top of your kidneys, spark into action and release a surge of the stress hormone cortisol. Quite often people can think they have kidney pain or backache, when it is in fact pain in the adrenal glands as they work away. Cortisol boosts your heart rate, elevates your blood pressure and increases your energy supply to help you to either stand and fight or make a run for it! That's what we are designed to do in a state of stress alert, run or fight! Did you know that? It is called the 'fight or flight' mechanism. Back in the caveman days, when we were sporting the sexy loin cloth, we would have either run as fast as our little legs could carry us in the opposite direction from the sabre toothed tiger or stood and fought it, bravely, to get a tasty meal - and stop us from being one!! The fight or flight action by our bodies is perfectly natural -and it is a great response, (life -saving on occasions!) providing our bodies are allowed to return to normal shortly afterwards. It is designed as a short term fix to a problem, (lasting minutes) rather than a long term state to be in - for example; carrying on for months on end - and that's where things can all go horribly wrong.

These days fighting a dinosaur is not what the stress response is about. Now it looks more like sitting on the motorway in a ten mile queue, meeting deadlines at work, being placed on musical hold on the telephone(grrrrr....), running the kids around to fit in their busy social diaries, juggling finances, looking after needy relatives, working towards exams, being bullied at school or work, being a new mum, loneliness, unemployment, exposure to cold, environmental toxins, pain, too much exercise, dealing with a severe illness or watching your favourite football team play badly or....Wow! The list is endless! I am sure you could write your own list of all the stressors in your life if you gave it some thought and had enough paper!

Anyway, back to the explanation...... Once the adrenal glands are set into action they release the hormone cortisol, which increases sugars in the bloodstream, alters your immune systems responses and shuts down your digestive system, your reproductive system and growth system as your brain knows these are not a priority at this moment in time. Did you understand that? Your amazing body shuts down the systems that it can survive without in the short term so that it can give you energy to deal with the stress. I am going to repeat the fact that the systems shut down - just to make sure you are getting this – that's the digestive, the reproductive and the growth systems. The problem is that if your stress is long term and not short term, these systems remain shut down, or partially shut down in the long term too. Are you beginning to see how stress has an impact on your health? Do you see why stress may be the reason you suffer indigestion, lack of sex drive or infertility?

An interesting fact here – stress creates diarrhoea, why? Because when under stress your body is designed to make you as light as possible so that you can run as fast as possible. Hence, a quick evacuation of any food that is weighing you down is on the cards. Now you know why you get a dodgy belly and need the loo fast when you are feeling nervous!

If you are in a constant state of stress, cortisol is released continually and your body is in shut down mode constantly too. This means all the basic functions, such as eating and digesting, can become really difficult – hence indigestion, heartburn, constipation, stomach cramps etc. Nutrients are not released into your body effectively if you are not digesting properly and even when they are, your internal transport system will not be working to full capacity (it will be on strike, part time, due to not getting a full pay of nutrients) which means that your vital organs will be starved of their basic lifesaving nutrients. This weakens your body, including your brain (it needs feeding too!). If your brain is affected your mental capacity to deal with stress will be reduced, and with a weakened body comes a weakened immune system, both of which will leave you wide open to mental and physical health issues. You become run down, lethargic, and bugged by colds, headaches, eczema, asthma, digestive issues, depression, poor memory, nervous irritability, elevated blood pressure, muscle and joint pain, insomnia, allergies and the threat of more serious health implications not so far off –for example, cancer, heart attack, stroke etc. . It's a downward spiral, my friend, which paints a very gloomy, but real picture.

Cortisol regulates metabolism of fats, proteins and carbohydrates. This has a direct impact on blood sugars and therefore a cortisol imbalance may become a precursor for diabetes and weight gain. If you have a few extra kilos which you cannot explain, (for example even if you eat healthily and exercise on a regular basis) the chances are your body is reacting to stress. Bit of a nasty one this stress thing isn't it? Just think, you are doing everything you can to be healthy and drop that inch or two – you are eating healthily and have joined the gym, yet still you can't squeeze into your skinny jeans and feel sexy.

The adrenal glands also produce DHEA, which is known as the fountain of youth hormone – they never call it a hormone in the movies do they? When this becomes affected you start to age quicker both on the exterior and on the interior! More wrinkles and an aged heart, not such good news. The fact is my friend, no matter how many face creams you purchase to combat your wrinkles, if your stress levels are high you are wasting your money! The best anti- aging product is not only free, but within your very own grasp. It is aptly called, 'Stress Management'.

Learning to deal with stress is the key not only to fewer wrinkles, but to damage limitation for your overall health. You cannot avoid stress, remember, it is there every single day, no matter who you are, what you do, how old you are or how wealthy you are! Recognizing it is the first step forward and then you can deal with it. Learning the skills of stress management will change your life and possibly even save it! It's time to take action to turn your stress into the positive attribute it can be, rather than a destructive menace.

There are many signs that you are suffering from too much stress. See if you can relate to any of these: Memory problems, an inability to concentrate, eating more or less than normal, sleeping too much, or suffering from insomnia. Feeling anxious, agitated or overwhelmed, being moody or short tempered. Suffering from digestive problems, stomach pains, frequent colds and infections. Having a rapid heartbeat or feeling dizzy or short of breath. Having a very low sex drive. Feeling out of sorts…but unable to put your finger on what is exactly wrong.

I could write a book purely on stress and stress management alone, and indeed there are many out there. However, 'The Wellbeing Touch - an uncomplicated guide to great health - naturally!' is designed as a simple approach to health and so I am going to give you six steps to follow so that you can begin to manage your stress successfully. But just before I do, I want to share with you an example of poor stress management, just so you get the picture:

One morning one of my clients, who we will know as Bert, opened a letter from a company that was asking him for money, whereas if the company had checked their records, they would have found they had already been paid. OK, annoying, irritating, time -wasting and frustrating, but not life threatening wouldn't you agree?

Poor Bert, who has blood pressure issues and is prone to strokes, didn't deal too well with the stress he felt due to this letter. Rather he acted without thought for his well- being and chose to go loopy, losing his temper and shouting down the telephone at the company for over 20 minutes. Heaven knows what his blood pressure was like for those 20 minutes! What did it gain him? Apparently Bert all but fainted, felt nausea and suffered pain in his chest. Great choice, wouldn't you agree, in exchange for a letter a possible heart attack! That's a letter, i.e. a piece of paper with black ink on it, hmmmm. For the rest of the day Bert felt like he had done 10 rounds with Mike Tyson, although it was just a telephone call to some nice lady in the company office (who was probably feeling the effects of stress too by the end of the telephone call)! Bert suffered an all -day headache and was unable to give his best at work, which is important to him. Another great exchange – a twenty minute telephone call for an all-day headache! Way to go Bert!

On a positive note, Bert did manage to get the problem sorted - there's always a silver lining - and Bert is still alive to tell the tale (double silver lining). But, at what possible cost to his health? The way he chose to handle this situation, meant it became life threatening for him (remember this was a piece of paper with black ink on it) and his reaction may well have caused internal damage. Instead of picking up the telephone in haste and anger, he could have given it some thought, taken a deep breath, judged how important is was in the grand scheme of things, realised that his payment had somehow merely been missed, responded in writing, or in a calm and controlled manner and gone on to have a great day.....without any negative impact to his health. Simple really, as I pointed out to him.....and he agreed! (And he felt a bit silly – well very silly actually.) Bert is now doing much better since he has learnt to follow my six basic rules of stress management, which if you too follow as a protocol, will give you a good, solid start for managing your stress.

Step 1 - Recognition.

The first rule is to recognise when you are under stress and what causes your stress. This is very personal, as what may be stressful to one person may not cause another to even blink.

Sit down and make a list of all the things that cause stress in your life – take your time and have plenty of paper to hand! When you see things written down the visualisation makes you more aware and helps you understand what causes your angst. Then you can deal with each stressor one at a time in a productive way. Writing a list may well demonstrate to you a pattern of the types of things you find stressful, making it easier to recognise future stressors when they appear.

The minute you feel something raise your stress levels, stop and think, 'Ahhh this is a stressor. I need to recognise it as one and follow the rules of dealing with it.' This means, before anything else, step back and breathe. Do not react – especially in the way poor Bert did!

You'll notice that your breathing patterns change throughout the day especially when you are stressed! Making them even again will bring a sense of calm. When your breathing is even, i.e. equal inhalation and exhalation, you become more present, focused and poised; and you are in a much more powerful state of being – you are back in control! You have heard many times I am sure people say, 'count to ten, count to ten!' when they are stressed well here is a little exercise and you only have to count to seven:

Sit still and be quiet (you can do this anywhere, even at work!). Settle into your position and breathe in through your nose for the count of seven. Then hold it for the count of seven before exhaling for the count of seven. Then hold it again for seven before repeating from the beginning. ...and relax....

Step 2 - Ground your stressor and down size it.

Ground it like you would a teenager when they do something you do not approve of. Take the wind out of its sails my friend. Ground the stress and then downsize it. A bit like throwing a piece of play dough on the table, rolling it into a ball and then splatting it into a pancake with your hand – which, incidentally, feels very good to do! When things bother you, you tend to blow them up out of all proportion by concentrating your mind continuously on them. You literally grow them! You need to bring them back down to size with a firm hand, and one that is in control (see the next step).

Going back to dear Bert, if you remember I referred to his stressor as a piece of paper with black ink on it. You may think that is belittling his life, but I see it as belittling the stress, and it was a piece of paper with black ink on it that caused him to raise his blood pressure to dangerous levels. A piece of paper – which, if I am correct in thinking, is in itself not a danger to anyone. You can do the same and turn complicated stressors into grounded challenges, of the right size, to be dealt with in a controlled manner and over –come in a calm, non -damaging way.

Step 3 – Control.

You are in control my friend. You sit in the driving seat of your life. You have the ability to allow stress to have Armageddon implications or merely tickle your toes. No stress is worth cancer, a heart attack, a stroke, pain or gross upset. This is stress management. This is saving your health and maybe your life. So obviously, this makes sense.

> Note here - If you are stressed your stomach acid can be low, so aid your digestion by squeezing a lemon over your food- or mix some lemon juice with olive oil to make a delicious and healthy dressing for fish or salad.

Going back to Bert again - it is a great example of how he had complete control over the stress. He literally held the control in his hands, but he chose to use the control in an unhelpful way.

Which raises the question – 'Why would you want to cause self-harm?' I am sure if some thug in the street approached you aggressively you would defend yourself; and if he punched you in the stomach and caused internal damage you would see him arrested and dealt with for the damage he caused you. I am sure if someone told you to jump off a third floor balcony to get your morning coffee, you would not because you know it would harm or kill you. We are born with self- preservation skills, but when it comes to dealing with stress, we forget to defend, throw those skills willy nilly off the balcony, and allow some thug at the bottom to punch them into the ground.

Remember you have the ability to control how you deal with whatever comes your way in the way you choose, so let it be one of benefit. Have confidence in yourself and your ability to influence events and persevere through challenges in a way that will be beneficial to you. Ask for help if you need it – this is still being in control! There will always be stressors in life that you can't do anything about so learn to accept the inevitable and go with the flow rather than push relentlessly against it.

Step 4 – Find the balance.

Once you recognise your stressor and realise that no matter how big or small the stress is, you have control over it, it is time to decide how you can deal calmly with the issue and in so doing cause as little damage to your health as possible, so that you can go ahead and have a lovely day (and life!).

> Here are two great questions us coaches use: 'What is the worst thing that could happen?' 'What is the best thing that could happen?' It is always good to ask yourself these questions and it could be beneficial to make a list. Remember there is always something good to come out of something bad.

Life is a balance my friend, and for every bad situation there will be a good side to it too. I know that may sound a little difficult to comprehend in certain situations, but it is true. Always look at the bigger picture. We do tend to suffer from tunnel vision, especially when things are not going quite to plan.

Once you have allowed your doom and gloom to come to a climax, take the same amount of time to find the silver lining – there is one, no matter how dire the situation seems at the time. You just need to take a closer look, like you would if you were given a dish of strange food and you were very hungry. I am sure you would repeatedly prod it about until you found something in it that you could eat. The same with your stressor, delve around a little until you find that tasty morsel.

When you find the balance it will take the sting out of the tail and you will begin to see that the situation it is not as utterly gloomy as you first thought. Sometimes, even, you may find that it is actually a really positive situation for you - and the whole thing will turn on its head. Take, for example, another client of mine, Abby Cadabby, who lost her job of 27 years because the company she was working for was down-sizing. Abby was devastated and thought life was not worth living anymore. After she had finished pouring out all her woes about her situation I smiled at her and said 'How fantastic for you Abby that now you are free to pursue your life dreams.' Dear Abby Cadabby was stunned by my response and sat with her mouth open. She was obviously thinking that I had either a) not listened to a word she had said, b) not understood a word she had said, or c) was in utter cloud cuckoo land. To be honest I was d) happy she had been given an opportunity to do something other than slave away for a company that obviously did not respect her services even after 27 years.

I took the time to explain to Abby Cadabby, over a much needed cup of tea, where I was going with my statement and eventually, and thankfully (otherwise I might have ended up wearing the tea) she got the idea. I am happy to say that now Abby runs her own cottage garden industry, which she absolutely loves and always dreamed of, but thought could never be more than a hobby. She makes good money, OK, a little less than what she was earning before, but she has not worked at this for 27 years yet!! All it took was a little stepping back, down-sizing of the stressor in line with the company she used to work for, positive control and balance. After consideration and a grounded mind,(rather than one that was leaping about and tearing it's hair out) Abby found the silver lining . That is so magic.

Step 5 – Action. Learn to act and not react!

You realise a stress is upon you, but you have wisely taken control and you have been very good and found the internal balance so you can be more calm. You have grounded and down sized your stressor, so now what are you going to do about it?

The way you take action now will have a huge bearing on what happens later. Think of Bert who bellowed down the telephone, not wise action even though it did get the problem sorted. He could still have got the result he wanted in a calm, non -damaging way. He reacted – and reactions often happen without thought.

Here is another example of a client's action that was not helpful in dealing with the situation – this is a 'bury my head in the sand and hope it goes away' situation – a man of no action! We will call him Ernie as we have Bert and I do love a bit of Ernie and Bert!

Ernie, a father of two in his early forties was suffering

from severe peeing problems that had been going on for six months, but he chose to do absolutely nothing about it, fearing it was something drastic. And so his problem grew until a very sick Ernie ended up in hospital in severe pain with kidney stones blocking his tubes. Ouch, ouch, ouch!!! The hospital sorted out the problem, but Ernie remained quite poorly and sore, (ouch again!) for a while afterwards. Furthermore he had not been working to full capacity before as his ill health was affecting his concentration and ability to give his all. Ernie suffered far more than he needed to. As a result of the' bury my head in the sand' approach, he had to take time out from work – never great when you are self- employed - lost a big contract, had to cancel the Euro Disney family trip (very unpopular with the small Ernies), fell behind on the mortgage, and had a few self-esteem issues after. But I am happy to report that Ernie is fine now and the Disney trip is happening next year (dad is back in favour again). We have worked on his self-esteem and he is back up there and business is going well again. But by not taking any action, it cost him lots, which it need not have done, as I pointed out to him. And just like Bert, Ernie felt a bit silly too!

People tend not to take action because of the feeling of FEAR. 'Bury my head in the sand' Ernie, was afraid of going to the doctor fearing he had something serious like cancer. He did have something that was seriously impairing his health, but because of his ungrounded fear, he allowed it to get to emergency levels. And what if he did have cancer? Was leaving it making the cancer better? By facing his fear he could have saved himself so much stress.

Fear is a feeling, like love and happiness. It is your own emotion which varies upon how you develop it inside your head. You can make a monster out of an ant if you fear it and imagine it a million times its size (bit like I do with spiders), and you can face your worst enemy if you see him for a human being the same as you (I always imagine my enemies in pyjamas or not managing stress!!!). Fear is made for you to walk through, as you can. The vast majority of our fears never come to pass.... remember that!

There is always a need to take action, even if that is allowing yourself to go with the flow, but action in a way that will be of benefit to you. It is not helpful to react and it is not helpful to bury your head in the sand. You can take some form of action whatever the nature of the situation. It is only you who will tie your own hands and believe there is nothing that can be done, or that the problem is too big for you to contend with – that is your thought and not your reality once grounded. There is always a way. Make a plan, draw up a course of action, using small steps if need be, ask for help if you need it, and slowly, and calmly, find the correct course of action. Remember you are your best friend, so don't give your best friend health issues to contend with on top of everything else.

Step 6 - Eat right!

Being in great physical shape places you a better position to deal with stress. How you eat and how you manage your health is paramount to beating the stress threat.

> Breakfast is the meal that can set your mood for the day. Eat high sugar content cereals, toast with jam or marmalade and your body will be challenged from the start with a blood sugar surge, giving you a spurt of energy and then dropping your mood and your energy like a stone. And talking of stones, these foods, which trigger a blood sugar spike will see your body releasing unnecessary cortisol that will turn to fat around your middle.

The most common action people take to help with their stress is to reach for high sugar foods, caffeine, alcohol and nicotine! Nooooo…(imagine me jumping through the air in slow motion wanting to save you from an attack by a jam doughnut). These things are just about the worst possible items to grab! Sadly the only help these substances bring is a quicker way to ensure adrenal collapse, which, trust me, will not help your stress! I know this from the personal experience I had when I was ill. I didn't know any better back then (I was up there with Ernie and Bert) and was grabbing Pro Plus tablets and extra bars of chocolate to get me through my days (Big Bird!). I felt I was too exhausted and stressed to make it through my day alone and without my 'fix'. After the initial ten minute pick me up, instead of helping, they dropped me like a stone and I would feel worse and worse and so I would reach for more. Even doing many hours of exercise a day, and eating my anorexic ant diet(apart from the chocolate) for the first time in my life, apart from during my pregnancies (when I was ENORMOUS), I was piling on weight which just did not make any sense . This upset me and stressed me out even further, so fuelling the self -defeating stress cycle. I was weakening my adrenal glands (the stress glands) with everything I did, until one day they collapsed and so did I. Not an experience I would wish on anyone.

Go back to the initial explanation of stress and review the way in which cortisol is involved in blood sugar. By eating or drinking or smoking things that will elevate the blood sugars further you will be enhancing the stress reaction. Indeed, even when you are in a state of calm, such stimulants do exactly that - they stimulate - and their affect is exacerbated under stress.

Certain foods can, however, soothe stress like a cold flannel on a hot head, and help you in your quest to manage it. Certain foods will help you regain control, which has got to be a plus in such situations! You need foods that can counteract the damage, which does not mean quick fix foods that often heighten the strain - so put down your family size bag of crisps! The diet I always advocate is quite simply, the one that nature has provided and not the one that humans have processed. It's low in sugar, salt, bad fats and refined carbs, but is high in vitamins, minerals, protein and healthy fats which all provide optimum nutrition and lower stress rates.

Slice up an avocado, a large tomato, and add some tuna/chicken/buffalo mozzarella and fresh basil leaves, drizzle with olive oil, add a little squeeze of lemon juice and munch away knowing you are feeding your body a stress control lunch.

Cut caffeine, nicotine, alcohol and sugar intake down, if not out. Yes I know you feel you need even more of these things when you are under stress but they are not your friends and will only stab you in the back. Follow the diet guide in my chapter 'The Balanced Diet' and you will feel much better and less stressed. In simple terms this means eating as much fresh unprocessed foods as you can and really bulking up on the vegetables! Eat regularly and not hastily and mindlessly. Drink plenty of water. Feed your body and feed your mind, then you will be in a healthier position to deal with what is on your plate (on your plate, get it?). If you are reaching for foods that will naturally starve your brain of nutrients and have a negative impact on your health, how can you expect yourself to respond well to stress? You will not have the power to do so......and this will stress you out even more!

Here are a few foods that really help in times of stress:

Prunes - Stress suppresses immunity levels and so extra antioxidants are needed. Prunes may not look pretty but are high on the ORAC scale – oxygen radical absorbency capacity – which is a measurement for how high a food is in antioxidants. Of course prunes have other great benefits too – they are great at getting things moving if you are a little bunged up – if you get what I mean?! Soak dried prunes in water over night and have for breakfast on some porridge, or some natural yogurt in the morning. If you like tinned prunes, try to have the ones in natural juice and not in syrup. Snack on a couple of dried prunes in the afternoon.

Almonds - Almonds are packed with magnesium,

which regulates the stress hormone cortisol. Magnesium deficiency (which is widespread amongst us) is also related to fatigue which can be exasperated by stress. Ground almonds are a superb addition to your morning smoothie, porridge or yogurt giving you a healthy start to your day. Almonds are a fabulous snack food - you could have some with your prunes! I love using ground almonds in place of flour when baking a cake. The cakes always taste more light and delicious.

Everything stops for tea, or it should, don't you agree? There is nothing quite like a cuppa is there my friend? Herbal and fruit teas are naturally caffeine free and this puts less pressure on the stress glands but black and fresh is equally as good – just beware of the caffeine content. There is certainly a relaxing comfort in a cup of tea, which, given the chance, will soothe away stress. Whilst you are drinking it, sit back for those two minutes (stop whatever you are doing!) and clear your mind – have yourself a real tea break! You can always spice tea up with slices of lemon, lime, orange, cinnamon or ginger - or a combination of some or all of these which will also have added health benefits. Try Chamomile with a dash of honey before bed, to aid restful sleep for instance.

Talking of fruit - Stress sucks away at your vitamin C levels, depleting your body of it, impairing your immune system and leaving you open to all manner of lurgies and bugs. Oranges, kiwis, cranberries, red and yellow peppers and tomatoes have a good amount of vitamin C in them and to make the best of all that natural Vitamin C eat them fresh and raw.

Eat protein rich foods such as eggs, meat, fish, cheese,

and beans, which are shown to satisfy hunger for longer and stabilise blood sugars, preventing mood swings and irritability. Here is one nutrient perhaps we could all do with a little bit more of - an amino acid, which you get from eating protein, known as Taurine. It supports insulin health, can prevent diabetes, elevates energy production, is a potent brain nutrient, lowers blood pressure, protects the heart, helps with detoxification, and fights inflammation – see what I mean!? Foods that are natural sources of Taurine are animal products such as seafood, meat, milk, and eggs.

Be inventive and make yourself a poached egg, on a little wilted or fresh spinach and a sprinkle of feta cheese on top for a super de-stress breakfast – yes greens for breakfast! This makes a great start to your day, supporting your immune system and blood sugars from the very beginning!

Your body has been designed for your stress hormone cortisol to fall in the evening so that you can rest and sleep like a baby. You need foods that aid this state of restfulness and not foods that stimulate you so that you lie there counting endless amounts of fluffy, white sheep all night. Slow release carbohydrates such as wild rice or brown basmati rice can regulate blood glucose levels during sleep so that you don't wake at all hours of the night. Walnuts are a good source of tryptophan, a sleep-enhancing amino acid that helps make serotonin and melatonin, the "body clock" hormone that sets your sleep-wake cycles. Turkey, lobster and prawns also contain tryptophan. Eat these with green leafy vegetables such as kale and spinach which, loaded with calcium, helps the brain use tryptophan to manufacture melatonin -your sleep enhancing friend.

> Knock up a turkey/prawn stir fry, sprinkled with walnuts for a restful supper, or make a yummy green vegetable soup and serve with a side of brown basmati rice drizzled with avocado oil. Both are quick, healthy suppers that will have you easing your cortisol down, 'til you are ready to dream away. .....

Chickpeas are also a good source of tryptophan, so a light, pre bedtime snack of hummus and oat cakes , which also help to stabilise blood sugars, could be a great way to head into a good night's sleep.

Eat your food mindfully. Think about what you are doing. Avoid eating on the go and switch off the TV so you pay more attention to what is going into your mouth! Take time, as always, to smell your food before you begin so that the enzymes necessary to digest your food, are released before the food enters your mouth. Chew well, as digestion begins in your mouth as you are about to find out!

Well, my friend, that's it. We have covered the six steps to help you get on the road for great stress management. Just think, once you get into the swing of things you too may be accused of not knowing what it is like to be under stress!

- Recognise stress,
- Ground it,
- Control it,
- Balance it,

- Act upon it,
- Eat right.

But just before we end this section on stress, here are two little extras, (value for money this e-book!) which if you practice may help you further with your stress management too. Firstly, take a walk. Get out in the fresh air and do what we as humans are designed to do....walk. It will help you to unwind, de stress and clear your thinking. Refer to the paragraph on walking in my chapter on exercise. Secondly, find time to relax. You do not need hours, although of course a weekend of relaxing or a week on holiday is absolutely marvellous! But if you do not have the luxury of such time, find ways at home to relax. Practice deep breathing (which of course, you could do anywhere), turn your bathroom into a mini spa with candles and soft music and lay in a warm bath, spend time with friends , visit an art exhibition, whatever it takes to help take your mind away from your stressors and relaxes you. Time out will leave you feeling refreshed and in a better, more composed position to cope and deal with what lies ahead of you.

Whatever you do, do not lie awake all night stressing and worrying. Turning into an insomniac will be of no help what so ever! From your bed, in your night attire, with your hair all back combed, there is nothing you can do to sort your problems. Nothing. Absolutely nothing!!!! It is far more beneficial to switch that mind of yours off, and have some sleep (there is a reason sleep deprivation is used as a form of torture). Only then will you have the power, energy and clear, alert thinking, to sort whatever challenges lie in your way. If you are affected by stress interfering with your sleep, stop accepting this is how it is, and find a way to return to a restful night's sleep. Trust me, my friend, life is a whole lot easier after a good sleep, and remember, we are all for life being as easy as possible!

Set the rules of stress management in motion and begin to see a difference in your health and your life. Do not leave stress unmanaged, but instead learn the art of stress management. Remember stress has serious side- effects. Whatever you do, don't be one to try them!

The Digestive system

"Western doctors are like poor plumbers. They treat a splashing tube by cleaning up the water. These plumbers are extremely apt at drying up the water, constantly inventing new, expensive, and refined methods of drying up water. Somebody should teach them how to close the tap."
— Denis Parsons Burkitt

Are you a poor plumber too? Perhaps you are one of the many who are constantly treating all kinds of health symptoms with indigestion remedies, laxatives, pain killers and decongestants? My friend, if you were to take a little time to look at, then treat the cause, rather than just addressing the symptoms, you too could turn off the tap. Supporting effective digestion, absorption and elimination is often the first step toward optimal health for many of my clients. Of course, there are many important steps to take to improve digestion, like working on diet and fluid intake, encouraging regular relaxation and exercise, making time for meals, reducing the impact of stress and correcting nutrient deficiencies, but getting the digestive system to work to optimum levels is always the best place to start with any health complaint.

For sure eating a well- balanced diet will enhance your chances of having fabulous health, but however great your diet is, if your digestive system is compromised you will not be absorbing the vital nutrients your body needs in order to be fit and healthy. The causes of malabsorption – the lack of absorption of nutrients from the diet, such as fats, protein, vitamins, minerals - can include a lack of stomach acid, bacterial overgrowth in the small intestines, deficient bile production, chronic inflammation of the small intestine from food sensitivities (it is estimated that 20% of the population has adverse reactions to food – not that many of them realise this) and rapid transit time -diarrhoea. So in order to squeeze the best nutrition possible out of our food, we need not only a healthy, balanced diet, but a digestive system that is in a healthy working order too. You are what you eat, but you are also what you absorb and what you do, or do not, manage to eliminate.

We have a body that is superior in design to any computer, car, mobile telephone, or sat nav system. It is an incredible feat of biological engineering. So before you marvel at your new smartphone, be conscious of the fact that you already have something far superior, your body! It is complex, yet simple and works incredibly hard for 24 hours a day doing a thousand different jobs (a bit like being a woman! Sorry, that was a bit sexist!). However you are unaware of most of what is going on because you do not see it. The only time you do become aware of it is when you do not feel so good, and you suddenly feel an ache or a pain, you get a cold, a spot, or a more debilitating sickness. Only then do you sit up and realise that something in your body is NOT working well. Taking great care of this wonderful invention should be at the top of the list – yet more often than not, you take your body for granted and do not give any thought to its care. Prevention is always better and easier than cure and taking care of the body you have been blessed with is the greatest step in preventative medicine. My friend, disease does not come out of nowhere, it lurks in dark corners waiting for your immune system to be weak and then, bang! In jumps disease.

> I am wise enough to listen to what my body tells me (something I have learnt to do). Sometimes it may take a few hours or a couple of days for me to stop still enough to listen and appreciate its nagging....but I get there. Can you tune into yours? Do you listen, or are you like the majority, and are either deaf to its cries or choose to ignore them?

In my humble opinion, which I am sure is shared by many a professional, it is within the digestive system that the beginning and the end of your health resides. That means the secret to a wonderful healthy life lies in protecting and nurturing your digestive system. Many of us today have digestive problems including reflux or heartburn, irritable bowel, bloating, constipation, diarrhoea, and colitis. In fact, stomach problems, such as the now notorious IBS (Irritable Bowel Syndrome), account for millions of doctor's visits and billions in health care costs. But digestive problems cause disease far beyond your little stomach. Normalising gut function is one of the most important things I do for my clients. A healthy digestive system means a healthier body.

Sadly, despite its important role in our health, all too often we tend to treat our digestive tract like one large refuge dump. We relentlessly throw in the wrong fats, processed foods, sugar and chemicals in the belief that it is OK to do so. (You just need to take a look in your bin at home to see what you have thrown into your stomach – Is yours full of empty crisp, cake, and chocolate wrappers, 'diet' drink cans or ready meal packs?) Disrespected and abused, still our digestive system soldiers on, doing its utmost to protect you from harm, working night and day fighting the various invaders that would cause you sickness and delivering whatever nutrients it can find to your cells to keep you alive. What a hero! Do you know of another that would fight so hard to keep you fit, well and alive? And what do you do to thank it, help it, protect it, nourish it and support its sterling efforts?

If your skin is bad or you have allergies, if you can't seem to lose weight, or you suffer from an autoimmune disease , if you struggle with fibromyalgia, arthritis, high cholesterol or have recurring headaches, the real reason may be that your gut is unhealthy. This may be true even if you have NEVER had any digestive complaints. Now that's food for thought!

People automatically think coughs, colds and the flu when any discussion turns to the immune system, but there are far more serious health issues related to your immunity such as cancer, so supporting the immune system has far reaching implications. It is a complicated system and the challenges to it are everywhere – in the air, on surfaces, in our food and drink – and you have no idea how hard it works EVERYDAY. Just by eating something slightly rancid, something full of sugar or by having some nice stranger sneeze over you on the aeroplane, or touching the light switch in the office, your immune system is instantly challenged and work begins to protect you without you having to give it a second thought. It is when your immune system becomes super challenged and your body does not give it the support it needs that it starts not to be able to cope. These challenges for your immunity lurk all around us and the correct diet, exercise, relaxation, stress control and keeping your attitude towards your life and health a positive one, all play supportive roles. 80% of your immune system resides in your gastrointestinal tract, so if yours has any defect from indigestion to constant bloating your immunity is compromised!

Here is a true yet fun client story for you: Kermit was sent to me by his wife (can only be Miss Piggy!) – as most of my male clients are! Miss Piggy was fed up of Kermit's IBS and all the uncomfortable symptoms Kermit was suffering from. It was beginning to affect Miss Piggy's life too as it was impacting their social life and, more importantly, she had had enough of Kermit's complaining! Kermit no longer wanted to go out for dinner in case his stomach became swollen like a balloon and he had a 'gas attack', as it had become known between them. Of course, although Miss Piggy was affected, Kermit too was miserable with his IBS. Like most of my male clients, Kermit was trying to ignore what was going on (although he was most unsuccessful at it as it was becoming impossible to ignore) and was sceptical about what my work entailed, even though he had seen a vast difference in Miss Piggy's health issues since she consulted with me. Dear Kermit thought I was some kind of hippy witch doctor.....which I am not, not that I hold anything against hippy witch doctors you understand! As I assured him, I was only interested in his diet and lifestyle so that I could help him gain the control and hopefully, bust the IBS and keep Miss Piggy happy. I was not about to chant spells or ask him to either.

It turned out that Kermit was somewhat blocked up – both in his intestines and in his sinuses. He ate a very carbohydrate rich diet and worked very long hours in the family business, often staying at work late in the evening. When he was working late he would grab a sandwich or a pie from the local supermarket for his dinner....and that was after a similar lunch and cereal and toast for breakfast. Plus there was the fact that Kermit nibbled away throughout the day on naughty biscuits from the business biscuit barrel. Vegetables seemed to only make an appearance at weekends! Kermit was also quite stressed by his working practice and that was fuelled by the fact that he felt so constantly tired which is no surprise on the diet he at.

So, I changed Kermit's diet, insisting he started his day with protein, such as an egg, or a bowl of porridge topped with some berries and nuts. Lunch was no longer to be a sandwich but either a salad or some soup with a side of protein such as cold chicken, or some cheese and olives, and, if he was working late, more salad or soup. Kermit nodded his head like he could deal with that with a little extra effort....Miss Piggy said absolutely he would! (It was very funny, but I had to do my best to keep a straight face.) Kermit also took a course of digestive enzymes, probiotics, omega 3 oils and a multi vitamin.

Then one evening, after four weeks, Kermit wandered into my office unexpectedly. He had not booked an appointment, but as I was without clients and packing up for the day, I asked him to take a seat and tell me what was wrong. He clasped his hands and looked down at them, and then raised his head and, I quote, said 'I really did not believe in what you did, because I did not understand it. I thought it was hocus pocus woman's nonsense. Sorry but I have to be honest. However, I am completely in your debt. My IBS seems to have disappeared. I have no pain and more energy. But what is most interesting, and what I really did not expect from any of this is my sinuses are clear. You are, however, responsible also for my wife's attitude of 'I told you so.''.' I grinned, of course, like the Cheshire Cat, and this time could not help but chuckle! Kermit continued to follow the diet and even cut back on his working hours to take up cycling...this I was most impressed with as it was on his own initiative. Having tasted what a healthier lifestyle could be like, he wanted the full Monty....and I bet Miss Piggy enjoyed that too!!!

There is a strong connection between what you eat, how well you absorb the nutrients from your food and the working order of your immune system. There are vital nutrients such as Vitamins A, B6, and C as well as minerals such as Selenium and Zinc which are critical to its support. On the other hand stress, under eating, being overweight, eating a diet high in processed foods, having a low intake of protein, being sleep deprived, and over exercising will all lower your immune response – which also includes your inflammatory response. This as we have already discussed, is vital to your health, something many people do not realise.

Your body is the vessel through which you will experience your life. If you nurture it, keep it well-nourished and fit, you will enjoy life to its full potential. However, if you neglect your body and fail to nourish it, slowly this will reflect in what you can do and achieve. So ditch the excuses, focus on the results you want and be prepared to make some changes.

From the time you became an adult you started to determine for yourself what you were going to eat. If you are lucky, and had health conscious parents, your taste buds would lean towards fruit and vegetables, and if you were less lucky your taste buds might have preferred biscuits, cakes, bread, sweets, and junk food. However day by day you determine your future health by how well you look after yourself. Yet many of us throw all kinds of rubbish at our digestive systems, and still expect them, naturally, to get on with the job and sort it without complaint. As you get older, my friend, your body starts to rebel against the poor nutritional choices you may have been making. You may just realise that when you crawl out of bed in the morning! Your body begins to assert its own wisdom, and it goes on strike!

Tell me seriously, if your boss kept throwing all the worst jobs in the business at you, day after day, relentless in approach, in the end would you not get a little fed up and start complaining? If your boss paid you badly for everything he expected of you, would you put in so much effort? If your boss didn't give you the correct tools to do the job, could you do it properly to the expected standard? And if your boss shut you in the basement which was damp, dark, and full of toxic chemicals in it, would you feel full of energy, motivated and able to give the very best performance? I am sure that if you had a boss like that you would probably say to yourself, and to the boss, 'stuff that for a game of soldiers (or words to that effect)!'

Think of your digestive system as the worker, and you the boss. Do you think it is fair to keep throwing the proverbial crap at it (like processed foods, fats, sugars, alcohol and drugs) and expect it to do a fine job? No of course not, you are a kind boss. And if you keep throwing bad food choices into your digestive system, what would you expect to get out of it? Surely not the finest health and tip top energy? Of course not, you are a realist, as well as a kind boss!

When you take your diet back to what nature intended for even just a week, something fantastic happens. By eating natural foods and giving your body a break from refined flour, caffeine, unhealthy fats and sugar, your body can shed some pounds of water retention and your energy levels can soar. You improve your digestion, stop feeling bloated and stop feeling congested! Can you imagine how fabulous you would feel if you did this for more than a week?

To understand something as complex as the digestive system and the impact it has upon our health, it is good to have a floor plan - or a blue print if you like - of the system from beginning to end. If that sounds as if this section is about to become incredibly scientific and complicated, rest assured I have no wish to blind you with science and I will do my best to take you from the beginning to the end just as if you were taking a fun ride from the top to the bottom of a very large, colourful, bumpy slide. I merely want you to understand what your digestive system consists of and what an awesome job it does, so you may be convinced to take a little more care of it.

A hundred million neurotransmitters line the length of the gut, approximately the same number found in the brain. More than 70% of the body's serotonin (feel good factor), IS MADE IN THE GUT, NOT THE BRAIN! (Must be why chocolate makes me feel soooooo happy!). Ask yourself, could it be your dodgy digestion that is causing you to feel down, sad or depressed!? And just to harp on about it, once again, remember the body mind connection thingy!

There you stand at the top of the bumpy slide with a huge beaming smile (Bit like the one I had after Kermit popped in to see me) that draws attention to your mouth – the home of saliva, teeth and tongue. Your mouth plays an important role in communication, but we are concentrating in this chapter on what happens when you put something in it, rather than what tends to come out of it. It is here that digestion starts, before you have even taken a bite. Just the smell of food triggers the salivary glands to secrete saliva which contains amylase, an enzyme that digests starch and so digestion begins. The teeth chew food to mechanically break it down and once it is has been masticated the tongue and muscles in the floor of the mouth propel the food into the pharynx, where swallowing takes place.

While we are talking about what goes into your mouth, if you think you are eating portions that are on the large size, like most of us do, swap your knife and fork for chopsticks. They will slow you down and as a result you will probably eat less. Just be strict with yourself – if you can't eat it with the chopsticks, no cheating, you have to leave it! Of course, you may already be an accomplished chopstick eater...in which case, way to go!

It is, as I have already said, in the mouth that digestion begins my friend, before you have even taken your first bite. However, it is also here that lack of digestion can happen too when you eat too fast, on the run, or without so much as smelling your food before you stuff it in. If you do not anticipate your food by smell and taste your saliva will not be produced, which means your mouth will not be expecting to go to work and will be caught unprepared (don't you just hate that when someone knocks on your door, uninvited, when you are in your worst chill out tracksuit bottoms and hair completely dishevelled?!). Then if you do not chew your food slowly, your digestion will be compromised as it will not have time to work on breaking the food down, which results in undigested starches going directly into the stomach....the beginning of so many digestive complaints. I know this may sound utterly ridiculous, but you should chew your food many times before you swallow it, slowly and mindfully. A bit like a cow chewing the cud – that will look good at the next office dinner! Ok, it may take you a wee bit longer to eat, and you do not need to make it as obvious as a cow chewing the cud, but as a result you may find that no longer do you suffer painful indigestion after. You may find you feel fuller more quickly, hence you will eat less – always a bonus! Nothing to lose (except perhaps a kilo or two) and a very easy, cost effective solution to your indigestion!

Try sitting in front of your food for a minute or two before you begin in order to get the digestive juices flowing. Once you have that mouth- watering feeling, then dig in but.....slowly! The grab and go culture we have initiated regarding eating food is responsible for many digestive complaints. Perhaps if you were to eat with more deliberation you would not have to keep reaching for the indigestion remedies, which in the long run may create exacerbated symptoms .....just a suggestion!

OK we are over the first bump of the slide and down a very short straight bit- the oesophagus which seems to have only one function – it connects the mouth to the stomach and therefore carries food between the two. It transports food by coordinated contractions of a muscular lining, which is an automatic response you are probably not aware of unless you swallow something too big, hot or cold! Then you notice it!!!At the ends of the oesophagus there are sphincter muscles that stop the food from re- entering the oesophagus or the mouth. These relax when swallowing and relax when you are having a good old burp, which is sometimes why you get a little reflux.

Time for another little story for you to smile at my friend: One evening I attended my (then) partner's colleague's dinner party, which was full of barristers, judges, Justices of the Peace and Queen's counsellors. Yes a table full of intellects and Queen's English! I was the odd one out, not being involved in the law at all, unless you counted a recent parking ticket, (although many years previously I had studied and passed my exams as a Legal Executive, a back -up career my mother insisted on when I was dancing – never used!) . So I was, for the most part, completely ignored and sat in virtual silence chewing the cud. I did my usual people watching of the guests around the table, whilst trying not to slurp too much fine wine in case anyone decided they could talk to me. I couldn't help but watch one rather rounded and red faced older man, who we shall know as Elmo. Elmo seemed very jolly (influenced, of course, by the wine) but I couldn't help notice how he kept trying to suffocate the desire to burp. The more the evening went on, the more Elmo struggled to suffocate the burp, becoming more and more red faced and his chin was virtually disappearing into his chest as he tried! In the end he let out one enormous belch! The table was thrown into silence, but having watched him all evening, I let out a childish giggle, which neatly took the attention away from the embarrassed Elmo as eyes turned to an even more embarrassed me! For what seemed like a lifetime, but was merely a few seconds I am sure, I sat there desperately searching my head for something clever to say. At last I chirped up with a little explanation (in a slightly high pitched nervous voice – read this next bit fast and in a high pitched voice to get a feel for how I blurted)) about burping, indigestion and how to solve it naturally rather than taking antacids as most people do, because, generally, older people, such as the discerning company around the table, were more than likely already low in stomach acid, rather than needing to kill off what little they had left. After I finished there was another pause full of silence and I sat there, without breathing, but with a rather strained half- smile on my face. I was desperately waiting for either everyone to, please, go back to ignoring me so I could breathe again, or at least someone say something…..Then, to my amazement, and relief, everyone wanted to talk to me and I was the most sort after guest at the dinner table! (Boy, did that feel good and I am sure I looked like a peacock in full display!) All manner of health issues of the legal beagles were thrown into advice seeking conversation. It turned out to be a very busy evening for me, and I was so pleased I had gone easy on the vino! I didn't even get the chance to eat dessert…or even turn it down as it probably had gluten in it anyway. Elmo asked my advice and even though he said he would not change his diet because his life was full of social dinners, he did take a course of probiotics and digestive enzymes. To date he keeps a supply of these in his pocket, although now, he says, he only needs them on occasions because his digestion is so much better, whereas he had been suffering after eating even the smallest meal. Elmo is the very essence of a happy client.

Enough frivolity, back to the slide, my friend, and we are off the straight and over the next bump as the oesophagus leads to the stomach which lies in the upper abdominal cavity just under the diaphragm. The stomach stores the food we eat and mixes it with enzymes and Hydrochloric acid that begin to break it down into a liquid mixture called chyme. The stomach has quite a cocktail of these digestive juices which makes for a very acidic, corrosive environment and in order to protect itself the stomach has a thick mucus lining.

The stomach contains a whole host of bacteria, however usually, it is the only the 'good' bacteria that can survive such an acidic environment. We need these helpful bacteria to produce vitamins such as those that belong to the B family. They act like an army with a large protective shield to save us from the bad guys. If, for whatever reason your good bacteria are compromised, the bad bacteria will hold a mutiny and find a way to take over and thrive.

A few causes of heartburn: Too much food which can cause pressure changes in the stomach so the food gets pushed back into the lower part of the oesophagus. Eating late at night or after exercise can also be seen as over eating by the stomach as cannot eating all day and then eating a large meal once a day. Being over- weight or pregnant or wearing tight clothes can place the stomach under pressure. Drinking too many caffeinated drinks such as coffee, tea or cola and eating/drinking too much chocolate which contains caffeine. Overeating refined carbohydrates such as sugars, breads, and pasta, especially if accompanied by a low fibre diet. Smoking can cause heartburn particularly during or before a meal.

Eating a diet that feeds you good bacteria and that feeds the good bacteria itself, has a number of health benefits such as improving digestion, boosting your immune system, producing vitamins, regulating hormones and, reducing the risk of serious disease such as cancer. So you can imagine what happens when the opposite is true – not having enough good bacteria and the often dire implications that this has health wise. Our increased use of vaccinations and antibiotics plus enhancements in hygiene, such as the use of the anti-bacteria cleaning products, have led to health improvements for many people. But, sadly, these same factors have dramatically changed the internal ecosystem of bacteria in our gut, and this has also had an impact on our health.

The most common type of bad bacteria in the stomach is one called Helicobacter Pylori (H.Pylori). This invades the protective mucus of the stomach causing inflammation and infection and if there for a long time, can cause ulcers. H.Pylori is a complete tyrant to get rid of and causes a lot of pain and distress! Other potentially harmful bacteria can include salmonella and E.coli. and we know how sick these can make us feel! The good bacteria come from two families, Lactobacillius and Bifodobacteria and it is from these two that your main defence army is set.

Still on our ride down the bumpy slide the next bump is the first part of your small intestine which is called the duodenum – yes I know we are getting a little scientific here, after I promised to keep it simple, apologies. However I thought you may like to know that it is here that your pancreas releases digestive juices rich in enzymes that break down fats, carbohydrates and protein. You release bile here too, stored in your gallbladder, into your duodenum which helps break down fat. So it is quite an important little part of your digestion and that's why I thought I should mention it. But here we go over this bump and onto the next straight…..

The small intestine has finger like protrusions called villi, which help the food move along (with a little help from the peristalsis movement, although its primary job in the small intestine is to mix the chyme rather than move it) and these villi have blood capillaries in them. It is as the food touches these villi that the nutrients are absorbed into the blood stream of the body. Sometimes these villi become damaged, which is what happens to those with Coeliac disease or gluten intolerance for instance (gluten acts like a glue and sticks the villi flat to the surface of the small intestine, hence blocking the absorption of nutrients and causing damage). If this is the case then you will become nutrient deficient and this has a knock on effect on your well-being.....slowly causing weakness and disease. It took the medical profession the best part of 26 years to discover I had coeliac disease! My digestion was always chronic and I still suffer on and off as a result. But I am now no longer starved of nutrients and am fit and healthy and able to nurture my system.

The best forms of food for increasing your good bacteria levels are live yogurt, cottage cheese, kefir, tofu, soya yogurt, wine, sauerkraut and sourbread. You can also supplement through the use of probiotics which, if they are good ones, will supply millions of friendly bacteria per shot!

Still sliding on down my friend....Your food, which, if you have the correct amount of digestive enzymes in your system, and have a functioning gall bladder, will have been digested well and will also continue to slide on down, now into the large intestine.

Your large intestine, the bottom part of your bowel, is a hollow tube and is where the waste products of eating are stored until they are emptied from the body. It is stacked wall to wall with bacteria, which is normal and healthy, but not if it is the wrong kind of bacteria. If it is full of those unfriendly little creatures you see on the toilet cleaner advertisements, then you are in serious trouble. However if it is full of those sweet little 'friendly' bacteria you see in the yogurt advertisements,(despite the fact that the majority of those yogurts will not provide you with very much friendly bacteria), then you will be laughing all the way to the bathroom and still be breathing enough to be laughing after too!

G lutamine is the primary fuel of the small intestine and important for the pancreas {which produces digestive enzymes) and the colon as well. When glutamine is deficient, the digestive system is impaired or damaged. Soothe a sore digestive tract with a glutamine supplement.

Your bowel needs to be kept in a healthy balance my friend, and when the balance tips in favour of the bad guys this is when your health is in serious trouble of being compromised. Your body, being the amazing machine it is, will give you signs, and causing an environmentally unfriendly stink in the bathroom is one sure sign that the balance is out and that you need to rectify it .Your bowel will also demonstrate to you that it is sick in other parts of your body too, because it is part of the whole of you, so you may have backache, or headaches, or feel zapped of energy or down in the dumps. Your body is inter=connected throughout, that is why I cannot stress enough how important it is to look at the whole picture and be holistic in your approach to knowing what is wrong with you.

Suffering from gas in the digestive tract can be uncomfortable, painful and very embarrassing. It is predominately made up of methane which can have a detrimental effect on the colon starving it of short chain fatty acids, a food it needs, for the lining, leaving it more prone to polyps and colon cancer eeeek! Here are just a handful of causes of too much gas: irritation to the intestinal lining – usually caused by eating a diet high in refined carbohydrates, excess salt, processed oils, caffeine, alcohol and sugar. Other causes are eating too much, nutrient and/or digestive enzyme deficiencies, food allergies/intolerances and intestinal bacteria imbalance.

Inside your large intestine there is a mucous lining which should be lovely clean and slippery, so that your waste food can be moved along to the very end and deposited neatly in your toilet. The sad fact is though, that this lush mucus lining tends to get damaged over the years and once this is damaged there seems to be a hold up in being able to move the contents along. It has been known for people to hold onto their food for as long as a month or two, or even for years. Oh my word can you imagine what that food must be like my friend? Ok, no, I accept you really do not want to imagine what it is like, especially if you are reading this whilst eating! It is a gross thought for the best of us. You can have a check of your own transit time by munching on some sweetcorn and checking when you see it reappear the other end. I know some may wince at that, but seriously it is an interesting experiment, which you do in the privacy of your own bathroom (well not eating the sweetcorn, you can sit at the table for that bit). See how long it takes to get from A to B and this may give you a clue as to the state of your bowel.

Spots on your face, in particular on the cheeks are the tell-tale sign of a sluggish digestive system and this build-up of toxins can not only cause you spots but can also make you feel lethargic, tired and irritable. When your body is not eliminating waste effectively it uses the skin as an outlet.

Your food does not just slip down the slippery slope of your large intestine to the exit like you would if you were on an oily mat flying down the bumpy slide. It is propelled by muscular spasms called peristalsis. Your large intestine is very long and goes up the right side of your body until it is under your right rib, across until it is under the left rib and then it drops down the left side of your body to the exit known as your rectum and anus. But then you knew that didn't you? Well, probably the last bit. You were, however, less likely to be aware that your bowel goes right up under your rib cage. Does this make sense now when you think of some of the pain you have been experiencing? Few people would blame their bowel for pain up under their ribs, and most people say they have stomach pain but more often than not it is the large intestine to blame. Like all muscles you need to keep the large intestine in great shape or even the peristalsis becomes disturbed and disrupted and the food that needs to be pushed out as waste becomes stuck and caught and begins to rot....and you know the rest.

The large intestine absorbs water from your body to help you have soft, easy bowel movements. If you are dehydrated, then bowel movements will be affected and you will become constipated - a bit like trying to go down the bumpy slide with treacle on the bottom of your mat. About 70% of the population has been shown to be dehydrated at any one time, so check you are drinking plenty of fluids each day. Aim for 1.5 litres of water, aside from your caffeinated tea and coffee.

Apple Cider Vinegar has long been regarded as a versatile health aid. It aids digestion and weight control, so use it in your everyday cooking. Apart from that it is a wonderful, non-chemical cleaner for your home, a great skin toner, good on abrasions and is a fabulous hair rinse when diluted with water! I like a teaspoon in a glass of sparkling water with a stick of cinnamon as a refreshing drink that also calms the digestive system. You can also pour a few drops into your bath water and then relax in it to help relieve IBS symptoms, or rub a little directly onto your stomach area, which will be absorbed and help relieve discomfort.

What you eat also affects the large intestine and a diet high in processed foods which lack natural fibre will have a direct bearing on the function and will clog up the pipes! Dietary fibre is generally obtained from plant foods – fruit and vegetables – and is part of the plant that is indigestible for man and so the body expels it. A typical diet of meat, dairy products, bread and refined flours are without fibre and will certainly slow down the process of elimination.

If your large intestine does not get enough water and fibre then your stools will become hard and dry and moving the stools along will be very difficult resulting in damage to the large intestine and straining when you are sitting on the loo. Maybe now you have time to read the newspaper whilst sitting there? And straining will bring its own list of nasty side effects, apart from finger nail marks on the side of the toilet seat, such as hernias, varicose veins (yes, bet you didn't know those were caused by your bowel movements did you???), hiatus hernias, diverticulitis and haemorrhoids. Hard dry stools which take longer to pass expose carcinogens (cancer causing substances) to the colonic surface and, sadly, this may increase your risk of colorectal cancer!!! All this from eating the wrong foods and not drinking enough fluids, which if you think about it, is within your power to rectify starting from now – have a glass of water!

Lack of exercise is one of the most common causes of constipation. You need to move in order to keep your intestines moving. In evolutionary terms, as we have already discussed, our bodies are set up to move every day – see the chapter on Exercise. Any kind of exercise tones up all parts of your body including your muscles, your heart, lungs and intestines. Exercise also decreases anxiety which can also contribute to constipation.

And so we zoom off the end of our bumpy slide. This is the part when the waste products from your body are neatly deposited from your rectum and anus into the toilet and flushed away. Yee ha! What a relief.

That's it. We have gone from the top of the digestive tract to the bottom in very simple and easy to understand terms. But there are two other organs in between that are very important for digestion and these are the liver, and the pancreas and, yes I know, you thought the hard part was over, but I just want to give you a brief look at both of these:

The pancreas secretes digestive enzymes into the duodenum, you remember that word? Of course you do. I was just checking to see if you have been paying attention! It is the first segment of the small intestine. These enzymes break down protein, fats, and carbohydrates. The pancreas is also responsible for releasing insulin, secreting it directly into the bloodstream. This is the main hormone for controlling the sugar in your blood.

> Pancreatic enzymes help digest proteins, fats, carbohydrates and all fat-soluble vitamins (E, A, K, and D). They have an overall anti-inflammatory action in the body. Keep in mind that if your body does not make adequate pancreatic enzymes, you will not adequately digest many nutrients. Different people will develop different nutrient deficiencies, thus symptoms can vary widely.

The liver has multiple functions, not least to keep you free of toxins, but its main function within the digestive system is to process the nutrients absorbed from the small intestine – providing you have kindly put some in there in the first place! Bile released from the liver plays an important role in digesting fat. It takes the raw materials absorbed by the intestine and makes all the various chemicals the body needs to function. The liver is an absolutely amazing organ that deserves plenty of respect and tender loving care for the work it does. This is why it is a great idea to give it a helping hand sometimes and follow a good detox plan to give your liver a clean and clear start. And here is a little extra information you may find interesting - If you want to lower your cholesterol, try cleansing your liver before you embark on cholesterol lowering drugs. If your liver is not burning up enough fat it will be depositing it in your arteries! Oh and if it is depositing it there, it could well decide to leave a little elsewhere too, like around your heart or on the tops of your thighs which is not exactly where you want to find it I am sure!

> Is it time you said to yourself, 'Right that is it. I am no longer going to put up with the way I feel, the extra weight I am carrying, the health issues that bug me every day. It's get real time. This is it buddy, I am not playing the victim anymore. I am going to sort this out. I am going to turn off the tap!'

So there you have it. Your digestive system bought to you in simple, easy to understand terms. Did you realise that you had such an awesome factory processing your food inside you? Even as you sit here reading this, your factory is in full flow. Like anything, this factory needs your personal attention and plenty of servicing to keep it in working order. The more you abuse it, the less it will function. If you have any digestive issues, no matter how small you think they are, your digestive system is telling you that it needs a service. If your car was coughing and spluttering I am sure you would put it in for a service! Even if you are one of the few that do not have digestive issues, but are unfortunate enough to suffer from other health issues, maybe it would benefit you to service your digestive system.

It is all very simple and uncomplicated at the end of the day. If you feed your gut quality fuel, it will serve you well and you will remain fit and healthy. If you give it trash it will begin to malfunction and breakdown and in so doing, starve your body of the vital nutrients it needs to keep you alive, and disease free. Take care of your food factory, the place where your health has a beginning and an end, and in return it will take care of you.

So here you are my friend, standing, no longer at the top of the bumpy slide, but instead at a fork in the road regarding your health. To one side is the road you have been travelling, or dragging yourself along, until now. If you continue down this same old road, doing exactly what you have been doing, things will continue exactly as they are. So ask yourself how do you think you will feel a week from now? A month? A year? How pleased will you be that you have chosen to continue down the same old path? Is this really the way you want to go?

Or do you want to change? If so, how about taking the other path? It involves a change of direction, a change in approach, a change in the way you are doing things. Change is always a little scary I know! But with a little bit of personal effort, maybe some professional advice and by initiating changes, step by step, ask yourself how different do you think your health (and, as a result, your life) will feel in a week's time? A month? A year?

I feel the need my friend, to follow the questions and end this chapter with a little rhyme my mother use to teach the children when she was the Nursery School Head. I am sure you will understand why!

Teaching her babies to fly one day
The mother bird sat on the wall.
But they were afraid as they wobbled and swayed
And cried that they might fall.
The mother bird said, 'You have wings like mine.
Be brave. You really must try.'
So they took one more peep,
And gave a big leap,
And found that they could fly!

A Balanced Diet – All that Delicious Food!

'Let nothing which can be treated by diet be treated by other means.'

— Maimonides

Food, glorious food! Hot sausage and mustard. While we're in the mood, cold jelly and custard. Do you know why we eat food? Contrary to popular belief, it is not down to how yummy it looks, smells or tastes, although I appreciate it is difficult to eat food that you find unappetising yet very easy to get that mouth- watering feeling when you are eyeing up the goodies in the bakery cabinets! The real reason we eat food is to fuel our body so that we may have life. Food supplies us with life giving nutrients my friend, needed by every part of our body to keep us alive. Quite simply, without food, we will die.

Many years ago, before I had mastered the art of cooking, I managed to produce (and I am still not sure how I managed to do this) some rather disgusting, green pasta, better known in the family as 'The Gunge.' Neither the look nor the smell was the least bit appetising and the taste was equally stomach churning Of course, we didn't eat it and the vote was for beans on toast!

Thus food is needed to keep us alive, but it is also very important to understand how different types of food impact on our nutritional status and therefore our health. Not all foods offer us nutritional benefit, no matter how delicious they may taste - and some foods may in fact cause us more harm than good. The food we eat, as I have said before, is the greatest way we have of controlling how fit and well we are. Food has the power to tip our health from good to bad or bad to good, so it is worth investing in the best possible diet we can in order to live a healthy life. But please, my friend, do not be like some of my clients who despair and believe that eating healthily means nibbling grass all day and having a plate full of tasteless foodstuffs. We have come a long way in the preparation of food, and master chefs now tickle our taste buds every day. Food is a sensation to be relished and healthy food is no different – except that it is good for you of course! It is all about balancing the right things in the right proportions and rediscovering how amazing 'good' food actually is.

Nutrition refers to the relationship with the food you eat to the health of your body. It is a subject I believe should be taught in schools so that we learn from a young age how nutrition plays a leading role in our life. It is probably the most important issue of human health over which we all have control. Learning how to nourish yourself deserves to take priority and it is not exactly complicated to do.

But first we need to get a little scientific (just a little bit I promise) about the food we eat my friend. Essential nutrients such as proteins, fats, carbohydrates, vitamins and minerals are needed for life to exist and we should get a daily dose of each from the food we eat. This very fact highlights the need to eat a varied diet, full of nutritionally rich food. A deficiency of even one of these nutrients may lead to defects in biological functioning resulting in sub-optimum health, disease and possibly even death. Each nutrient has its own role for example: proteins are beneficial for hormones, blood, enzymes, genes and skin. Carbohydrates are great for providing energy. Fats help brain function, sex hormones and the utilization of Vitamin D. Vitamins are necessary for cell signalling and regulating cell and tissue growth, fighting toxins and boosting the immune system. And finally, there are various minerals that are essential in order to activate thousands of enzyme reactions within the body.

There is another dimension to eating well, one which many people do not realise – and that is its role in pain. Apart from the prevention of ailments by eating a good diet, if you are unfortunate enough to suffer from pain, whether it is caused by cancer, arthritis, a sports injury, a headache or even the common cold, there is pain relief available just in what we consume. But, on the other hand, there is also the potential to cause inflammation and therefore pain by the foods you eat. If you are gluten intolerant for example, you may well have abdominal pain - caused by foods that contain gluten - or if you have arthritis the deadly nightshade family of vegetables – aubergines, tomatoes, peppers and potatoes – may well be irritating the inflammation in your joints. Sugar alone is responsible for plenty of inflammation within the body. However, always looking on the bright side of life, there are healing foods such as ginger that has anti-inflammatory qualities, essential fats, such as those found in oily fish, which have anti-inflammatory qualities, and hot chillies which contain a substance called capsaicin, which can block the nerves power to transmit pain messages. The bright yellow spice, Turmeric has been shown to be similarly as effective as anti-inflammatory drugs, without the side effects! So we have the ability to eat a diet that will reduce pain, or a diet that will enhance pain's powers.

Clementine came to see me about her very inflamed digestive system which seemed to be sensitive to nearly every food she ate. (Clementine is not alone. Intolerant bowels are rife!) She also had rheumatoid arthritis in her spine, hips and hands which was crippling her and making life a tiring struggle. We removed the deadly nightshade family of vegetables, wheat and cow's milk from her diet, made a plan for her to eat six small meals a day made up of only three varieties of food at each mealtime, and introduced a high concentration supplement of turmeric and ginger, which also contained some vitamins and minerals, plus an Omega 3 fish oil. After one month Clementine's digestion had improved immensely and she was able to eat a greater variety of foodstuffs, providing she still treated her system with care. The pain from the arthritis had almost disappeared and the everyday chores of life, like dressing herself, was now much easier to do, rather than a painful struggle that she often needed help with. There is a huge link between an upset digestive system, the food you eat and arthritis, (and eczema and asthma) so repairing a damaged gut and altering the diet to compliment the health issue will inevitably have a direct impact on arthritic pain. And adding good anti-inflammatories such as turmeric, ginger and Omega 3 will ease inflammation and therefore pain throughout the body.

The food you munch through each day will have a bearing on the energy you have too. Perhaps my friend, you one of the many people who feel tired all the time? How many people do we both know who press the snooze button on the alarm clock over and over again before dragging themselves out of bed? And come afternoon, who would like a sneaky forty winks? Reach for the wrong food choices and your energy will have you up and down on a roller-coaster ride! If you want to feel well rested, alert and with a stable balance of energy throughout your day, you need the foods that offer great nutrients so that you will not suffer from sub-optimal cellular energy metabolism, resulting in feeling tired, lethargic and sluggish. Vegetables, beans, nuts, seeds, fruits, whole grains and quality animal protein all offer the body the best way to combat feelings of fatigue. Sadly, foods made from refined grains and lots of sugar, such as the majority of breakfast cereals, biscuits, white bread and pies, only guarantee you will continue to feel tired.

The food you eat will also play a vital role in your mood, thinking, and memory. Keeping your brain fed with a diet that is high in quality nutrients will keep it in much better shape than feeding it junk. If you expect your brain to perform to optimum levels, then it is important you feed it a diet of optimum nutrition. The brain is part of the body and just like all the cells of all other organs, brain cells are continually being renewed. Tomorrow's cells are therefore made up of what we eat today - which should make you think - or will what you ate yesterday not allow you to think today? In particular, when we are talking about the state of your mind the Omega 3 fats play a significant role, so a diet that is low in the essential Omega 3 fats will result in a mind that will not function how one would like. Research has shown that when Omega 3s are eliminated from diet, behaviour becomes anxious and stressful, learning becomes more difficult and mood becomes depressed. Today the consumption of Omega 3s in the Western world may be less than half what it was before the Second World War and curiously it is precisely since that period that depression has shown to be rising!

Pop a salmon steak or two onto a sheet of tin foil. Drizzle a little cider vinegar, a pinch of cumin, a pinch of coriander, some lemon juice and the zest of one lemon over the steaks. Fold the foil into a parcel and cook in the oven on 180 degrees for approximately 25-30 minutes, depending on the thickness of your salmon steaks. Serve with a rocket and spring onion salad and some sweet potato mash. If you can, cook enough salmon to have some cold for your lunch the following day.

I am sure that when you go to the supermarket to do your weekly shop my friend, you don't usually do this with a view to thinking about the foods you need to heal yourself this week! Or what foods you need to iron out your wrinkles, stabilise your energy or give your brain a boost. Barely a third of us shop for food with health in mind and about the same proportion of people does not know what the daily recommended amount of fruit and vegetables is. And even for those who do, many will not meet this goal on a regular basis. (By the way you should aim for your 8 a day....5 a day is a bare minimum and why would you want to skimp on good health?) Now is as good a time as any to explore and understand the super healing properties of food and to uncover the foods that can have a negative effect on your health too, so that you can establish a fabulous balanced diet for yourself. Food, glorious food! Hot sausage and mustard. While we're in the mood, cold jelly and custard. Do you know why we eat food? Contrary to popular belief, it is not down to how yummy it looks, smells or tastes, although I appreciate it is difficult to eat food that you find unappetising yet very easy to get that mouth- watering feeling when you are eyeing up the goodies in the bakery cabinets! The real reason we eat food is to fuel our body so that we may have life. Food supplies us with life giving nutrients my friend, needed by every part of our body to keep us alive. Quite simply, without food, we will die.

Thus food is needed to keep us alive, but it is also very important to understand how different types of food impact on our nutritional status and therefore our health. Not all foods offer us nutritional benefit, no matter how delicious they may taste - and some foods may in fact cause us more harm than good. The food we eat, as I have said before, is the greatest way we have of controlling how fit and well we are. Food has the power to tip our health from good to bad or bad to good, so it is worth investing in the best possible diet we can in order to live a healthy life. But please, my friend, do not be like some of my clients who despair and believe that eating healthily means nibbling grass all day and having a plate full of tasteless foodstuffs. We have come a long way in the preparation of food, and master chefs now tickle our taste buds every day. Food is a sensation to be relished and healthy food is no different – except that it is good for you of course! It is all about balancing the right things in the right proportions and rediscovering how amazing 'good' food actually is.

Nutrition refers to the relationship with the food you eat to the health of your body. It is a subject I believe should be taught in schools so that we learn from a young age how nutrition plays a leading role in our life. It is probably the most important issue of human health over which we all have control. Learning how to nourish yourself deserves to take priority and it is not exactly complicated to do.

But first we need to get a little scientific (just a little bit I promise) about the food we eat my friend: Essential nutrients such as proteins, fats, carbohydrates, vitamins and minerals are needed for life to exist and we should get a daily dose of each from the food we eat. This very fact highlights the need to eat a varied diet, full of nutritionally rich food. A deficiency of even one of these nutrients may lead to defects in biological functioning resulting in sub-optimum health, disease and possibly even death. Each nutrient has its own role for example: proteins are beneficial for hormones, blood, enzymes, genes and skin. Carbohydrates are great for providing energy. Fats help brain function, sex hormones and the utilization of Vitamin D. Vitamins are necessary for cell signalling and regulating cell and tissue growth, fighting toxins and boosting the immune system. And finally, there are various minerals that are essential in order to activate thousands of enzyme reactions within the body.

There is another dimension to eating well, one which many people do not realise – and that is its role in pain. Apart from the prevention of ailments by eating a good diet, if you are unfortunate enough to suffer from pain, whether it is caused by cancer, arthritis, a sports injury, a headache or even the common cold, there is pain relief available just in what we consume. But, on the other hand, there is also the potential to cause inflammation and therefore pain by the foods you eat. If you are gluten intolerant for example, you may well have abdominal pain - caused by foods that contain gluten - or if you have arthritis the deadly nightshade family of vegetables – aubergines, tomatoes, peppers and potatoes – may well be irritating the inflammation in your joints. Sugar alone is responsible for plenty of inflammation within the body. However, always looking on the bright side of life, there are healing foods such as ginger that has anti-inflammatory qualities, essential fats, such as those found in oily fish, which have anti-inflammatory qualities, and hot chillies which contain a substance called capsaicin, which can block the nerves power to transmit pain messages. The bright yellow spice, Turmeric has been shown to be similarly as effective as anti-inflammatory drugs, without the side effects! So we have the ability to eat a diet that will reduce pain, or a diet that will enhance pain's powers!

Clementine came to see me about her very inflamed digestive system which seemed to be sensitive to nearly every food she ate. (Clementine is not alone. Intolerant bowels are rife!) She also had rheumatoid arthritis in her spine, hips and hands which was crippling her and making life a tiring struggle. We removed the deadly nightshade family of vegetables, wheat and cow's milk from her diet, made a plan for her to eat six small meals a day made up of only three varieties of food at each mealtime, and introduced a high concentration supplement of turmeric and ginger, which also contained some vitamins and minerals, plus an Omega 3 fish oil. After one month Clementine's digestion had improved immensely and she was able to eat a greater variety of foodstuffs, providing she still treated her system with care. The pain from the arthritis had almost disappeared and the everyday chores of life, like dressing herself, was now much easier to do, rather than a painful struggle that she often needed help with. There is a huge link between an upset digestive system, the food you eat and arthritis, (and eczema and asthma) so repairing a damaged gut and altering the diet to compliment the health issue will inevitably have a direct impact on arthritic pain. And adding good anti-inflammatories such as turmeric, ginger and Omega 3 will ease inflammation and therefore pain throughout the body.

The food you munch through each day will have a bearing on the energy you have too. Perhaps my friend, you one of the many people who feel tired all the time? How many people do we both know who press the snooze button on the alarm clock over and over again before dragging themselves out of bed? And come afternoon, who would like a sneaky forty winks? Reach for the wrong food choices and your energy will have you up and down on a roller-coaster ride! If you want to feel well rested, alert and with a stable balance of energy throughout your day, you need the foods that offer great nutrients so that you will not suffer from sub-optimal cellular energy metabolism, resulting in feeling tired, lethargic and sluggish. Vegetables, beans, nuts, seeds, fruits, whole grains and quality animal protein all offer the body the best way to combat feelings of fatigue. Sadly, foods made from refined grains and lots of sugar, such as the majority of breakfast cereals, biscuits, white bread and pies, only guarantee you will continue to feel tired.

The food you eat will also play a vital role in your mood, thinking, and memory. Keeping your brain fed with a diet that is high in quality nutrients will keep it in much better shape than feeding it junk. If you expect your brain to perform to optimum levels, then it is important you feed it a diet of optimum nutrition. The brain is part of the body and just like all the cells of all other organs, brain cells are continually being renewed. Tomorrow's cells are therefore made up of what we eat today - which should make you think - or will what you ate yesterday not allow you to think today? In particular, when we are talking about the state of your mind the Omega 3 fats play a significant role, so a diet that is low in the essential Omega 3 fats will result in a mind that will not function how one would like. Research has shown that when Omega 3s are eliminated from diet, behaviour becomes anxious and stressful, learning becomes more difficult and mood becomes depressed. Today the consumption of Omega 3s in the Western world may be less than half what it was before the Second World War and curiously it is precisely since that period that depression has shown to be rising!

I am sure that when you go to the supermarket to do your weekly shop my friend, you don't usually do this with a view to thinking about the foods you need to heal yourself this week! Or what foods you need to iron out your wrinkles, stabilise your energy or give your brain a boost. Barely a third of us shop for food with health in mind and about the same proportion of people does not know what the daily recommended amount of fruit and vegetables is. And even for those who do, many will not meet this goal on a regular basis. (By the way you should aim for your 8 a day....5 a day is a bare minimum and why would you want to skimp on good health?) Now is as good a time as any to explore and understand the super healing properties of food and to uncover the foods that can have a negative effect on your health too, so that you can establish a fabulous balanced diet for yourself.

> Ginger root is great for travel and morning sickness and green olives help prevent motion sickness. So it sounds like a cocktail of water with slices of ginger, and an olive if you are going on your travels!

Everyone's nutritional needs are unique and depend on a whole host of factors, from the strengths and weaknesses you were born with, your present state of health, to the effects your current environment have on you. There is no single style of diet that tops them all, and your preferences count, but balanced eating is the first step to super nutritional healing and a life of abundant energy. As Hippocrates said, "Let food be thy medicine and medicine be thy food." Herbs, vegetables, fruits and nuts provided our first healing medicines and they still can, and do. Food is often your best remedy and your safest - you would find it difficult to overdose on parsley, or celery, I am sure!

> I am a great believer that for every ailment, nature has provided a cure....we just have to be clever enough to find it!
>
> For example: Carrot soup can cure diarrhoea as carrots contain balanced amounts of sodium and potassium, two electrolytes that a dehydrated stomach needs!

In evolutionary terms we have not had a very long time in which to have developed the capacity to eat, digest, benefit from and eliminate the processed foods on offer these days. Coping with foods that have changed in the last fifty years has left us wide open to all kinds of health issues as our bodies struggle to know what to do with them. There are many diseases these days that have their origins in the food we eat and lifestyles we lead, which without the intervention of modern medicine, would see the death rate of the modern world soar.

When we were running around in loin cloths we did not have such diseases and were more likely to die from falling ,breaking our limbs, getting infections from open wounds or being eaten by a wild beast. We were stronger back then, healthier and leaner and our food was what we hunted and gathered. We ate with the seasons and we walked or ran to gather or kill each day. We didn't eat vast amounts each day of the week, indeed some days we would have eaten very little or not at all. We would not have eaten a huge variety at each meal and may well have eaten just berries, or just wild boar, or just a fish. The fruit and vegetables would have been harvested and eaten the same day. There were no artificial growing methods, no herbicides or pesticides, and foodstuffs were not stored for months on end or being shipped half way around the world. The meat would have been fresh kill too, and from stock untouched by artificial growth hormones and antibiotics. We rarely cooked our food in those days and would therefore have benefited from the enzymes present in raw food, rather than killing the enzymes during the cooking process. We were able to make the most of what nature offered without any laboratory interference.

Enzymes are important as catalysts for regenerating, restoring and protecting us. There are over 3,000 in our bodies and they are responsible for kick- starting the chemical reactions involved in reproduction, breathing, digestion, growth, healing and combat against disease. So nutrients containing beneficial enzymes can have extremely positive consequences for our health! Raw vegetables and fruit are the best sources.

Alice Snuffleupagus is my very best friend (if we had gone to school together we would have been separated in the classroom, such are the giggles we share). Sadly poor Alice suffers from Crohn's disease - a long-term condition that causes inflammation of the lining of the digestive system from the mouth to the back passage, but most commonly in the last section of the small intestine (ileum) or the large intestine (colon). I advised Alice that due to her having Crohn's she was more than likely gluten intolerant and that it would probably benefit her health if she went without dairy too. I urged her to give up the grain and reduce her dairy intake. At first she went through the deprivation period, the detox healing crisis and the 'what else CAN I eat?' syndrome; but with gentle nurturing, books to read, diet sheets made uniquely for her, delicious homemade soups full of vitamins and minerals, no gluten, and limited dairy the results have been remarkable. Alice's malabsorption was chronic, and her stomach discomfort and bowel irregularities were painful, annoying and life altering. Gluten acts like a glue or papier-mâché in terms of what it does to the villi of the intestinal lining – flattening it and thus reducing its ability to absorb nutrients; now imagine how that must feel combined with the damage caused to the intestines by the Crohn's itself. However, just by eliminating gluten alone, Alice began to feel different. She found she no longer suffered the continual discomfort, or toilet sessions and it became very clear that her intestines started to increase absorption of the essential nutrients! Her hair condition changed, her skin became more radiant, she began to have colour in her cheeks, rather than the whiter than white look she normally sported. Her weight began to drop and her energy levels raised – she even found herself whizzing round her home with a duster before the school run, something she had not been able to achieve in years. As Alice's overall health improved, so did her eyesight and her reading glasses are now being recycled. She no longer needs the steroids handed out by the hospital, which in itself is an enormous boost to Alice's wellbeing – not least because the steroids had very negative effects on her general health and made her feel very depressed. Alice Snuffleupagus is on a major build up programme of all the vital nutrients and she understands the need for continual investment in her health. Furthermore, she recognises that there has to be a continual personal effort to maintain the control over the Crohn's Disease. But now she has the feeling that she is 'normal' again, Alice is more than happy to continue down this path as her future looks brighter and her present is a whole lot healthier and discomfort free than her recent past. And so the giggles go on!

How about a lovely bunch of coconuts? The health benefits of coconut derived products are vast: including increased energy, weight loss, natural antibiotic activity, thyroid balance, cholesterol reduction and insulin stabilisation. Try cooking with coconut oil. The fatty acids in the oil are 90% saturated, which makes coconut oil highly resistant to oxidation at high heats and therefore the perfect oil for high-heat cooking methods like frying. Coconut flour is gluten free, and makes very fine cakes! Coconut milk is delicious to cook with and as a milk alternative for your tea and coffee try a product called Koko.

As you are serious about improving your health, (I am assuming this is the case because you are reading this!) it's a good idea to take a long, hard look at your eating habits. When you're younger, your body has such vast reserves of energy that you can normally get away with poor food choices (although it is so much better to eat healthily from the start!) and continue to function well. It's as your body gets older that it starts to rebel, and the problems that have been caused from a nutrient poor diet begin to show.

I am sure you have heard and read many times that you should 'eat a balanced diet', and of course that is what I have been harping on about 'til now, but do you know what a balanced diet is? On average, you will spend around six years of your life eating. It would be six years well spent if it keeps you fit and healthy! A balanced diet will be one that offers you the best possible intake of nutrients for your body and brain so that both can be as healthy as possible. And as you clearly want to live a healthy life my friend, (I am making assumptions again!) with oodles of energy and without disease, it goes without saying that you need to nourish your body with the nutrients it requires to ensure you can do this.

The rewards of eating a diet that enhances your nutrient supply rather than depleting it (oh yes, eating certain foods can actually deplete your nutrient supply!) are many. You will have clearer skin, a sharper mind, a slimmer body, less coughs and colds, trouble free digestion (no IBS!!!), a better mood, less hormonal disruption, more energy and less overall illness. What fantastic perks of the job – the job being to ensure you eat correctly. It takes a little personal effort my friend, but it is an investment into you, an investment worth its weight in gold.

You have a choice and control over what you eat. You

can put the correct fuel into your tank or you can run it on fuel that will have it coughing and spluttering until it decides to give up the ghost. Your choice, as I said, but I am sure you would not, deliberately, put the wrong fuel into your car , so why would you choose to treat yourself any differently? I had a friend who was unfortunate enough to put the wrong fuel into a car (maybe he had not eaten enough essential Omega 3s!). It was extremely costly to reverse the damage, plus very time consuming and very stressful – especially as the car was not his! Ouch! Much the same with your body, making the wrong choices can be very costly, time consuming and stressful, only I see your body as a far more valuable machine than your car – you too I presume? Disease is draining on all aspects of life from physical energy to financial state, from family relationships to social life, from the fun you should be having to the success you should be achieving. Health, on the other hand, should bring with it a wonderful life.

Without having studied nutrition, which might I add your doctor may not have done in any depth, it is understandably difficult to see the wood from the trees with all the conflicting information out there regarding food and what to eat. It seems that each week there is yet another damming argument about a food that was previously thought of as healthy – which you have been munching away on believing you are doing a fine job by consuming! Plus there are the foods which you were lead to believe were unhealthy, which are now on the 'essential for good health' list. It can all become a rather confusing, messy bowl of information for which, my friend, you have my sympathy! But fear not, Big Bird is here, keeping it all as uncomplicated as possible, so that you may have the basics of a balanced diet under your belt, literally, and giving you well informed foundations to build on.

First let's drop the food bomb - achieving a 'perfect' diet is somewhat of a myth these days, and no matter how hard you try, you are probably falling short somewhere along the line. This is not entirely your fault, as food is not the same as it used to be and has become a highly processed commodity. Processed foods are sometimes even labelled as healthy, which can be very misleading, so go easy on yourself with any blame game. You know, fundamentally we thrive on natural plants and animals, but the marketing industry have distorted this somewhat to make us believe other things!

Many of our fruit and vegetables are grown in nutrient deficient soils due to over farming and the use of chemicals in pesticides and herbicides, which result in nutrient deficient produce. On top of that fruit and vegetables are often stored for months on end in cold storage and then lined up under artificial lights in the supermarkets, destroying any beneficial health properties they originally had. Maybe they have been grown using intensive farm methods and flown half way round the world to get to your local supermarket, which does not lean towards great nutrient content in the produce once it finally arrives. Most commercial meat and dairy is produced with the use of hormones and antibiotics to boost quick growth and continual production, resulting in a large amount of antibiotics and hormones being passed directly from animal to consumer.

Grains are pumped up using more and more of the indigestible gluten, and stripped of their goodness (and bleached) when processed into 'white' goods. Quite a sad and disturbing reality when one thinks about it. What once held the promise of a good nutritional diet has become a nutritionally insufficient one, shaken and not stirred into a cocktail which contains added chemicals, hormones and antibiotics.

However, people still tend to talk about eating this illusive 'perfect' diet, and often ask me if this is what I eat. I have to admit that a perfect diet is very hard to achieve even for me; however, I aim to have a balanced diet which is a little easier, and this will be our focus.

There are few of us in this world (although the number is growing) who know, believe and understand how food influences every aspect of health from migraines to asthma, PCOS (Poly Cystic Ovary Syndrome) to cancer, IBS to depression and Diabetes to strokes. Whatever your health issue, the food you eat or do not eat will have a bearing on it. It is a sad fact, that still many conventional doctors fail to recognise the importance of diet, although to me it is so basic – food is your fuel for life after all!

So, Big Bird, do tell,' What is a balanced diet?'

A balanced diet is not just about eating enough fruit and vegetables, although they play a major role in our dietary needs as you already know. A balanced diet is one that complements your overall lifestyle, genetic weaknesses and the environment you live in. We are all uniquely different, just look around you to see how each of us differs from the other, and as such we all have our own unique need for a different balance of nutrients. For example the nutrients needed by a growing child will differ from a person who is elderly. When you are pregnant you will need extra nutrients to help the unborn child to develop and to keep mum in good shape. If you are very active you will need more nutrients than the person who is quite inactive. What is balanced nutritionally for one person, may not be balanced for another. It's a bit like the' one size fits all' line of clothes – now that is a laugh isn't it!?

I am sure you are aware of the old saying 'You are what you eat', and this is very true up to a point, but even more so you are what you digest and absorb, including chemicals, pesticides and toxins. This is the difficult bit. Even environmental factors need to be considered when choosing your specific balanced diet. For example- factors such as cigarette smoke, exhaust fumes and general air pollution. For instance, if you are a cigarette smoker you will need to boost yourself with plenty of vitamin C as smoking robs the body of this vital immune supporting nutrient.

I am sorry if this is beginning to sound as if it may get a little complicated, especially as I have promised an uncomplicated way forward for you, but, rest assured I will do my best to keep things as simple as I can. Remember this book is designed to get you on the road to greater health, but, as I do not know you personally, and this book is meant for the millions, I cannot write down your unique diet for you. However, what is very important for now, is that we lay the foundations so that you are better informed to go further, healthily. You can do a great deal to influence your health positively by following the advice in this book and should you wish for the more personal touch you can consult with me via www.thewellbeingtouch. com

> By changing my clients diets and lifestyles I have eliminated bad moods, brought back periods, reduced stubborn weight issues, cleared up digestive upsets, improved complexions, installed energy, reversed diabetes type 2, reduced blood pressure and cholesterol , increased libido, controlled MS, boosted thyroid stimulation, enhanced fertility, banished aches and pains, and seen many come off of long term medication. Impressive- yes?

Many diet fads have come and gone which eliminate food groups – especially fats and carbs. This is possibly all well and good, but our engines are complicated, designed to run on a combination of fuels. A little of everything does you good, too much of one thing and not enough of another will tip the scales and result in your body being out of balance.

In simplistic language that means a balanced diet consists of pure, unadulterated meat, fish, legumes, nuts, seeds, fruit, vegetables, eggs, whole grains, and water. Maybe a little dairy......(we will talk dairy later!). There are some people who claim that we are better off without grains and legumes, as we have not had enough evolutionary years for our bodies to be able to digest them. However, in order to give you greater foodie options, I will leave them in this uncomplicated guide. I am also in two minds as to whether we are all better off without them or not and believe again, that it is down to each unique individual's tolerance.

A few years ago I visited a doctor for a 'new patient' check-up as I had moved areas. The doctor asked me why I did not eat gluten. I told her to refer to her records to see that I had Coeliac disease (where the immune system reacts abnormally to gluten -a protein found in wheat, rye, barley and oats-, causing small bowel damage). I was shocked by her response as she told me to go and eat some proper bread, as all the gluten free food stuff was nothing but hype! She continued to tell me there was nothing like having a nice cream bun with your morning coffee! I could see from her size where she was coming from! Needless to say, I found a different doctor's practice to join.

We should eat what nature has provided in the form it has provided for us in – good, healthy natural food that has contributed to our successful evolution. We were not meant to eat additives, preservatives, e numbers, saturated fats, copious amounts of sugar, salt and all those other unhelpful ingredients that are added to processed foods. We were meant to keep food natural and eat it as such.

Natural foods do NOT have an extensive ingredients list. A chicken, should read –Ingredients: Chicken. Nuts should read – Ingredients: Nuts. And so on. Anything with an ingredient list has been processed. Take a look on the back of packs next time you shop, you may be surprised or horrified at what is in your seemingly, natural food selection.

However the multi million pound food industry of today has complicated things – just what are they like??? They have worked as hard as they can to take away your need to think about where your food originated from and how it has landed itself in the nice packaging in front of you. No longer do you need to prepare your food from scratch or to experiment with herbs and spices. Now the taste comes in the form of added salts, fats and sugars, all surplus and often detrimental to our health. Why have we allowed the chef experience and the social circle of eating to disappear from our daily lives?

No need to worry as the processed food industry has it all covered! These companies have clever marketing campaigns that tell you 'You want it, need it, and love it'. You are also told that certain products will save you time and money, that you can eat on the run, and have great food in minutes….. and you believe it…..why wouldn't you? This is probably because we have been told not to question what the experts say and we have decided not to be curious about what is being thrown down our throats! But these industries are experts in making money, and not particularly interested in preserving your health – why should they be? And after all, as I have already stated, your health is your own responsibility. Possibly the biggest issue created by the processed food companies is the opportunity for us to be lazy when it comes to our diet.

Processed foods are, in my opinion, the scourge of the food industry. Packed full of fat, salt, and hidden sugars, with some of the worst offenders being those labelled as 'diet foods' -these foods can be highly toxic to your system. Have you ever wondered why you wake up the next morning after a take away or a microwaveable dinner, frozen pizza, or some of those noodle things in pots, feeling sluggish, lethargic, puffy, and grumpy? They disrupt the balance of your blood sugars, your body's salt reserves and fat deposits and give you zero in the way of beneficial nutrients. They are, what we refer to as, empty calorie food, i.e. they are full of calories with zero nutrient value! So what is the point of eating them?

When you eat processed foods, not only do you fail to provide any real nutrients for your body to work with, but you also burden it with the difficult task of eliminating the rubbish you have chosen to consume. By having to eliminate this food your body will use up a lot of energy, which in turn will zap it from another place where it is needed. As a result you begin to become run down and fatigued as your immune system and other vital systems become starved of energy.

If the reason you eat is to fuel your body so you can have a turbo charged day, what is the point of eating foods with such negative health values? The answer my friend, lies all in the taste. Yep, that's it...you like the taste. That's the point, the whole point and nothing but the point to these destructive foods. We have forgotten how fantastic unprocessed food can taste, without the added salts, sugars, fats etc. that our taste buds have become accustomed to. And this is because we have forgotten how to cook simple nutritious food for ourselves.

I was just thinking maybe I was a little harsh on processed foods saying that the only point was the taste. Of course there is another point and that is convenience! It saves you time and effort, well so you think. OK again, I give in on the 6 minute microwave meal, that is pretty quick, but you could knock yourself up a delicious, nutritious salad in that time. (Before you start slating salad for being boring and tasteless, if you slam a few lettuce leaves, a tomato and a slice of cucumber on a plate, I might agree, but if you REALLY make a salad it can be an absolute taste sensation).

Try some of these easy to make salads....

Rocket, and spinach salad, with warm mushrooms and cherry tomatoes gently sautéed in garlic and olive oil, topped with a chicken/tuna fillet.

or

Green, red and yellow pepper strips with prawns, lambs lettuce and sliced avocado, tossed in avocado oil and balsamic vinegar.

or

Roasted Butternut Squash with the skin on and cubed, crumbled feta, rocket, pine nuts, fresh rosemary and olive oil.

or

Chopped cos lettuce, diced cucumber, chopped spring onions and sliced radishes mixed in a dressing of tahini, cumin, crushed garlic and olive oil and sprinkled with dried paprika.

How about a bowl of homemade soup? Some soups you can make in a flash, others you could prepare a batch for the week and then just reheat in a couple of minutes, so beating the 6 minute microwave toxic load!

Watercress soup

Watercress is packed with the nutrients calcium, iron, and folate and cancer protective isothiocyanates, making it a true super food. This is a really quick and easy soup that tastes delicious.

1 chopped onion
1 or 2 crushed garlic cloves (according to taste),
1 can of green lentils or chickpeas (for protein)
1 litre vegetable stock
150g watercress

Heat some olive/coconut oil in a pan and fry the onions and garlic for 5 minutes. Add the lentils/chickpeas and stock and simmer for 15 minutes. Remove from the heat, add the watercress and blitz in a blender until smooth whilst adding seasoning to taste. Serve topped with a little crumbled feta cheese or pumpkin seeds on top.

Consider the fact that processed food that tastes good and is convenient at the time that you are eating it may actually cost you more time in the future when you are sick, having to visit the doctor, hospital, enduring cancer treatment programs, or being in a kidney dialysis unit….and then it is really expensive and not just in time! Point put over….have you got it?

I helped the Cookie Monster, who came to me complaining about a lack of energy, a slow metabolism, too much weight and depression. I asked the Cookie Monster to be very honest with me about the diet he ate on a daily basis. When I ask my clients this question, I know that a good 50% of those in front of me do not answer entirely honestly. Sweet really, but I normally catch them out! Anyway, I asked the Cookie Monster to be very honest with me and bless him, he was. He ate chocolate éclairs for breakfast, a cheese sandwich from the local garage and a bag of crisps and a slice of chocolate cheesecake for lunch, some more chocolate éclairs for an afternoon snack and a microwave dinner for supper. He was a processed food garbage deposit. It was easy to help the Cookie Monster get better once I managed to persuade him to completely change his diet. I persuaded him to start cooking vegetables and eating fruit, meat, fish, nuts and well balanced, but easy meals (eating healthily does not mean slaving for endless hours in a kitchen). The Cookie Monster thought he had a major illness when he came to me. He did in a way - processed food-itis! Poor Cookie Monster was really sick, but he was fortunate not be suffering from any major diseases, although if he had carried on eating in the same way, he may well have become ill later on. As it was, his whole being was run down. He looked and felt very ill, was weak, and didn't have a positive thought in his mind. After we changed his diet the Cookie Monster was a different person altogether. His energy soared, he lost about three stone in weight, and he said he had never felt happier or more on top of life. The Cookie Monster vowed he would never touch processed food stuffs again as long as he lived. I am sure having felt such a huge difference, he never will. Om nom nom nom.

I recently encouraged Count Von Count to give up sugar. He found his tea and coffee to be very odd at first having always added two teaspoons of sugar to each cup, but after just three days told me he could actually taste the tea and the coffee and said that it tasted amazing! All that natural flavour had been masked and killed by his sugar hit. Once Count Von Count realised that he was giving up at least eight teaspoons a day of sugar in his drinks alone, and he worked out how much that amounted to over a year, and over the years he had been consuming it, he was even more committed to giving up his addiction which was, of course, the reason behind many health issues that were bugging him. He loved the fact that he found taste again. He also loved the fact that his frequent headaches disappeared, and his mood lifted!

Many children with Attention Deficit Disorder respond well to a diet that is low in sugar and supplemented with essential fats.

Whilst we are on the subject of sugar, I want to have a little word with you about it, my friend. This is just in case you did not know the effect sugar has upon your body, despite the high profile it has received in the media recently. Sugar – pure, white and deadly! (That's a nice dramatic statement!) In years gone past we would have consumed about a pound of sugar a year....nowadays it is over 100 pounds a year, (eeeek!!!!) which is one massive increase! My friend there is no denying the fact that, and I am not going to sugar coat this for you, sugar is BAD for your health. Are you addicted? Probably, yes. I had a client some years ago who actually found it easier to kick her heroin addiction than to quit sugar. I think that says a whole lot about sugar!

Every time something with sugar touches your taste buds it triggers the pancreas to send out a lot of insulin to break down and use the sugar. Because sugar is burned very quickly, you are left with a very high amount of insulin in the blood. This free roaming insulin causes you to crave more sugary foods and so the vicious cycle begins. The sugar will raise your energy levels sharply, but then will drop you back down like a stone leaving you feeling lethargic and tired. So what happens next? You will grab some more to lift you back up again and so the cycle continues! Any wonder we have an obesity crisis?

We all know that too much sugar in the diet causes obesity, diabetes (which is the fastest growing disease of this century), nutrient deficiencies and, dental problems – and dental issues are one of the leading causes of seeking medical help for children in the UK. Excess sugar contributes to premature ageing, and too many other serious diseases. However, despite our best efforts to cut back, the amount we consume has actually increased. Why has this happened? Probably because the sugar we consume is a hidden ingredient in the processed foods that we buy. A fact we do not necessarily realise when we are buying these foods.

Read the ingredient labels on the foods you buy, preferably before you buy them and have a sort through the foodstuffs in your cupboards. Sugar is one of the food industry's top ingredients. It's used to brown, preserve, thicken, aerate, stabilise, sweeten and bulk out our foods and is in everything from 'health snacks', diet foods and yogurts through to breads, processed meats, sauces, dressings, baby formula, drinks, crisps and pizzas.

Any sugar added to a diet, other than that already present in fruit and vegetables is – believe it or not- too much sugar for you to handle! We are just not designed to have it in our system. So whether it be a teaspoon in your morning coffee, a juicy cream cake, or a ready microwave meal, it is too much sugar and will be a burden on your body, with the potential to make you sick! Believe me, those who eat a diet high in sugar will always be the ones suffering from recurrent coughs, colds and other illnesses. Sugar has a devastating effect on the immune system.

Checking the labels of these foods may be a bit of a pain at first but you'll soon get used to doing it- and you are likely to get some surprises! You may well be shocked by how much sugar you are actually consuming. Look for the 'Carbohydrates (of which sugars)' in the nutrition information panel on the labels. 10g sugar or more per 100g is a whole load of sugar!! 2g sugar or less per 100g is a better amount. Even when you are reading the labels sometimes it is difficult to decipher how much sugar is in a food as they are only required to give you the `total grams` of sugar on the content label. If you see sugar (or any of the other names for sugar as listed below) itemised within the first few ingredients or itemised several times within the list, you'll know that the product is likely to be full of sugar, and, hence, best avoided.

Sugar, by any other name, is still a sugar, but it can be so well disguised.

Brown sugar, Confectioner's sugar, Granulated sugar, Sucrose, Fructose, Glucose , Dextrose, Galactose, Lactose, Maltose, Invert sugar, Raw sugar, Corn syrup, High-fructose corn syrup, Honey, Maple syrup, Molasses, Hydrolysed starch.

High Fructose corn syrup (HFCS) is an ingredient in almost every processed or sweetened food going from fizzy drinks to biscuits, cakes, breakfast cereals and canned foods. You will even find it in some soups, crackers, and yogurt! (This is very much the edited list) Once HFCS enters the cell it becomes acetyl-CoA which is made into cholesterol, produces a fatty liver and slows down your metabolism. Not a health food then this HFCS! Well, not a good health food, let's put it that way! Watch out for it and avoid it if you can.

Back to processed foods - I was a classic example of being caught in the marketing trap of ' diet foods', another multi million pound food industry that may well have you fooled into believing is a great way to go! ***Note to oneself: No matter what the title of the food is, If it's packaged, it's probably loaded with sugar.*** Always battling to keep my weight as low as possible as I danced, I would opt for the low fat options of everything. I had no idea how that by doing this I was starving my body of the essential fats I needed to fuel my highly energetic lifestyle and failing to ensure the inflammation within my body caused by the constant bombardment of exercise, was kept under control. I also did not understand that you still need to eat fat to remain slim. Furthermore I had not grasped the fact that these low fat foods contain many hidden sugars that will a) make you fat and b) cause other health issues. Now I understand and have learnt from my mistakes, but I had to pay for them first. So hopefully by reading this, dear friend, I will have saved you from making similar mistakes. Funnily enough, my mother told me to stop eating the diet food rubbish, as she called it, and just eat normally. She was right as she invariably and annoyingly is! Shame I did not listen to her (and not just about the food either!).

Any low- fat product can be harmful. When the low-fat guidelines first came out, all the major food manufacturers thought it would be a great and profitable idea to make food stuffs that were 'reduced fat', or 'fat free'. They wanted to jump on the band wagon and bring 'healthy' low-fat foods to the supermarket shelves, (and make a bomb!) in order to sell to those who had suddenly become health/ fat conscious. However, when fat has been removed from food, there is a big problem – namely that the food lacks flavour. For this reason, the food manufacturers add sugar which is, of course, not a fat, it's a carbohydrate. Therefore, a product can be labelled "low fat", leading you to believe it is good for you, even though it is loaded with sugar (and therefore actually fattening) and not so good for your health. Low fat foods are a bit of a gimmick and they have just one benefit - they make their manufacturers millions and billions as you fall victim to the marketing blurb!

I humbly apologise but talking about sugar is now

going to get me going about another favourite gripe of mine - the artificial sweetener. Are you one of the millions who use artificial sweeteners under the illusion that they are better for you than sugar? As far as artificial sweeteners are concerned, manufacturers have successfully convinced millions of us, the mega- trusting public, that the chemicals used in artificially sweetened products are safe and better for our waistline. Always good to know that chemicals are good for us! But think about it, if you're consuming a food or beverage created in a laboratory, as the artificial sweetener is, instead of by nature, your body isn't designed to recognise it, true? It is a foreign substance and as a foreign substance it may cause short-term and long-lasting health problems, placing an additional strain on your body.

Some artificial sweeteners have been referred to as 'known carcinogens', meaning they are poisonous and could cause cancer! They are known to cause brain damage, depression, MS like symptoms and many other horrible illnesses and so it is best to avoid artificial sweeteners – how have they ever been allowed to be introduced into our foods? In small amounts, these substances are not harmful, or so they say, but anyone can exceed the small amount by eating what they think is healthy food – for example, diet soft drinks and diet yoghurts. Depending on the quantities you consume, you could experience the following side effects after consuming a large quantity of artificial sweetener: Upset stomach, sugar cravings, mood swings, increased fat around your middle, problems sleeping.

Rosita came to me with continual daily headaches. Rosita had been to many specialists who were scanning her for brain tumours, the lot. She was having such a bad time, not just with the headaches, but with the terrible upset of not knowing what was wrong with her and if she was going to die. In our consultation Rosita cried continually and I was really moved. However, I noticed she chewed gum, all time she was talking to me. I asked her if she always chewed gum (really I was thinking it was a wee bit impolite), and she said she chewed every day, all the time and had done for years. But she informed me, it was sugar free gum, so it was kind to her teeth and waistline. It was as if a giant light bulb had suddenly been switched on in my head – complete with a full orchestral 'der der da der'! After a very hard two hour consultation, to Rosita's surprise, I simply recommended she stopped the gum for a week. After a day she had major detox symptoms, for example her headaches were worse, and she was on my back complaining BIG time!!!!..... but after five days, she had fewer headaches and by day ten, none at all! We then sorted the rest of her diet and stress out and she was discharged from the hospital because they could find nothing wrong with her. The medics never confirmed my theory, but never opposed it either. Rosita was convinced it was the gum, and it was only her opinion that mattered in the end.

Could there be a connection between your health issues and artificial sweeteners? Again, do your own research and you will see how these artificial sweeteners are not quite the healthy products you may believe. As I always say to my clients, opt for the full fat stuff and nothing labelled as a 'diet' food, or sugar free or low fat, as they have been artificially sweetened. Eat what nature has kindly provided for you, not what has been chemically produced. We have not reached a time yet, on our planet that we have to rely on food created in a lab because the land has stopped producing......and I hope we never will!

There is another little demon hiding in your processed foods – salt. We all need salt to stay fit and healthy. It's made up of sodium chloride and we need sodium, along with potassium, to help carry the electrical impulses that control our bodily functions. However, it is the correct ratio of sodium to potassium that we need for these chemical reactions to work properly. When not in the right ratio, salt causes high blood pressure and strains the kidneys. Salt can also damage the brain and the high salt intake is linked to vascular dementia. This means that arteries to your brain get clogged and this may lead to a stroke. Think about that as you shake it all over! There is another reason to watch your salt intake - sugar and bad fats are blamed for the weight issues so many people suffer from, and with great justification I may add. However salt also plays its part! That innocent white crystal causes water retention, which may give you a few extra pounds and inches.

Enough about sugar and salt, let's get stuck into dairy (which is processed too really) and why I have reservations about it. Milk is promoted as healthy, vital for babies, full of active proteins for adults and essential for those at risk from osteoporosis, true? You are repeatedly told on the TV advertisements that you need these products for your little ones to develop strong bones and to prevent your grandmother from not healing after breaking her arm. True again? If you were to believe all the advertising you could be forgiven for believing that you could end up a bendy mess on the floor if you were to ever go without milk! However, cow's milk is not intended for consumption by any other animal other than baby cows. Would you suckle a cow? No, didn't think so. And would you see a cow suckle a pig? Of course not. I mean, think about this seriously for one minute my friend, are humans the same size and build as a cow? Fortunately not, or getting into the car to go to work may be a bit of an issue. So why would we drink the milk intended to grow a calf into a cow? We humans are the only breed on this planet who believes that consuming the milk of another species is a good idea – eh derrrr. You see, if compared, the profile of nutrients of cow's milk with that of human milk shows major differences. Cow's milk contains about three times as much protein as human milk and about as much as four times the amount of calcium, both of which can place excessive burdens on the human kidneys. The ratio is so different that it has the potential to make us sick. Many, many people are intolerant to cow's milk too, and it plays havoc in their body – they just do not realise it!

As a little passing thought, we would be much better off if we ditched the cow's milk and went back to suckling our mothers, after all, their milk IS meant for human consumption. Don't fancy that? Didn't think you would. Perhaps we could bottle it instead of suckling it? Nice drop of breast milk in your morning tea. Still not tempted? That's because after you have been weaned, it is meant to be the end of your milk consumption! Period!

The largest animals that wander our planet such as elephants and hippopotamuses, and even cows, are all vegans – well they eat plants. Which means that they get their wonderful, huge, strong bones from the calcium contained in plants…..they do not need to suckle milk from a different species! Eat your greens my friend and you will have plenty of calcium, in the right ratio for your body to use successfully!

It is not my wish to worry you my friend, but the dairy story goes on….Over the years, as is the case with most of our foods, the quality of dairy products has changed and not always for the better. It is also the case that we now consume way too much (great when we are not meant to consume it in the first place). It has been calculated that in the UK dairy consumption per week is about the same as the amount of petrol we put in our cars – around 5 litres. This is incredible if you think about it! The real worrying thing about this is that milk products now supply a high percentage of female sex steroids such as oestrogen and progesterone in the diet. Significant concentrations of the male hormone testosterone also occur in cheese, milk and milk derived products. Because hormones have such important roles, the levels of hormones in our bodies are carefully controlled. But eat too much dairy and the added hormones are passed onto us, and are in excess to those we have naturally in our bodies, so knocking out the careful balance. Particular concern has been expressed about the oestrogen content of cow's milk. By consuming these products you will be consuming also the extra hormones, which, you really do not need in order to stay in good health. Any wonder why there are so many hormonal issues these days? The next time someone you know is suffering from a real bad dose of Pre Menstrual Tension, maybe it will be worth getting them to give up the white stuff.

And here is the real bomb shell my friend- part of the role of hormones is to help control when and how often cells multiply. Changes in hormone levels, such as when we consume too much dairy that has had hormones added, can interfere with this process and that, my friend, can lead to cancer.

Personally I stay well away from anything produced by a cow, and consume only goat or sheep cheese in small amounts, and no animal milk whatsoever. It would be very rare to see me eat yogurt, but if I did it would be from goat or sheep and not from cow.   Goat and sheep produce tend to be less tampered with than the produce from cows. I honestly cringe when I see people downing their huge morning lattes, full fat or that watery stuff they call skimmed, and wonder if these people have hormonal issues - like irregular/painful periods, mood swings, or fertility issues, let alone their potential risk of exacerbating a genetic predisposition to hormonal cancer - such as breast, womb or prostate. If you are genetically pre disposed to hormonal cancers or have had a brush with them, do yourself an enormous preventative favour and stay away from dairy, in particular cow's produce. Likewise, if you suffer with hormonal issues, stay away from dairy, again in particular cow's produce.

My own experience has shown that consuming cow's produce creates breast lumps – sore and painful ones at that! Enough to keep me well away. If you feel you want to indulge, be careful and limit your amount. By the way, it makes no difference whether it is full fat milk or skimmed, it is still milk from another species and therefore not intended for you!!! If you really enjoy your milk and cannot imagine life without it (although life without it is easy and healthy) try some of the many milk alternatives now available, such as almond/hazelnut/rice or , a favourite of mine, coconut milk. Research this subject of hormonal cancers and dairy on your own, it is enough to put you off when you do! Like anything, uncovering the real facts by yourself can be eye opening and life changing.

OK my friend, I think that is enough griping about food, after all we want to have a positive attitude towards it rather than one of dread. As a nutritionist it wouldn't be right if I neglected to tell you about the food that is not good for you, but I also want to encourage you to eat, not put you off, so gripe over!

Let's turn our attention now to how we eat. How do you prepare and eat your food? Do you have a quick fix attitude to your food? Are you always eating in a hurry, running whilst chomping down a sandwich, or throwing together a quick meal for the family? If so, slow down. You will be missing out on the enjoyment of food and will be eating purely for the sake of it, without any real thought about what you are eating. Food should be lingered over and enjoyed with family or friends. At least sit back and eat with intention and focus on the fact that you are eating! Become mindful of what you are doing. Aside from anything else, digestion begins in the mouth, so if you are swallowing down your food without chewing it properly you are missing out on the first stage of digestion. Result – indigestion! And we are back to undigested food in our body, which does not paint a pretty picture of good health. Take a few moments to actually look at your food before you put it in your mouth. Allow the salivary glands to work, which will release the digestive enzymes ready to break down your food. Ask yourself if your choice of food is going to heal or harm you. If you realise it could cause you harm ask yourself if you really want to it eat. If you do, go ahead and eat and do so without reproach. But if you decide you do not want it, leave it and reach for a healthier choice.

Eat when you are hungry, not just when the clock says it is time to eat. It really baffles, well annoys me actually, when I am in the UK and want to eat lunch at 3pm, and find that restaurants stop serving at 2! Apparently there are certain hours you can feel hungry between, after that....well you just did not conform! This attitude of 'eating when the clock says', or 'lunch MUST be between twelve and two' is a form of programming which takes away our ability to decide for ourselves if and when we need to eat. Have we lost our ability to know when we are hungry? Were we more intelligent when we were babies and announced with a loud yell when our little bodies told us we were hungry? I am not convinced that we screamed between twelve and two each day for lunch back then...but ask your mother!! If you are not hungry my friend, try not to just stuff your face because it is time to, wait until you are hungry, or just eat something small. Of course, I understand and also promote, that if you have blood sugar problems it has been demonstrated that eating small amounts, regularly, help to stabilise your blood sugars. You know yourself better than I know you, so you need to take responsibility and master the correct balance of eating.

Here's a little gem of information that may surprise you -I am not a breakfast eater and it is rare that I partake; despite all the fuss about the so called importance of breakfast (could this be just another ploy to get you to buy cereal?). I am sure that statement was enough to raise some eyebrows, especially as I am a nutritionist, and isn't it the job of such to promote the importance of breakfast???!! Well, I have a different way of thinking. I tend to eat when I am hungry and not, when I am not, and I am rarely hungry early in the morning. Even when I am staying in the best of hotels, with the most delicious breakfast buffet laid out in front of me, I will rarely have anything (no discount on the room rate though!). Some days I will go until 3pm before I eat, other days it is 11am, depending on when my body tells me that I am hungry. When it does, I listen to it and eat (unless I am in the UK looking for a restaurant at 2.05pm!). Also when I feel I have had enough, and that is before I am stuffed like a Christmas turkey, I stop eating! (I am a fan of the 80/20 rule - eat until you are 80% full and leave the other 20% of space for digestion.)The only clock I obey, is my own body clock. I know I am fortunate not to work in an environment where your breaks for food and drinks are set, but even if you do, listen to how hungry you are and eat accordingly. Do your best to 'tune in' to your body and ignore the clock on the wall! And make sure you are eating because you are hungry and not because you are bored or thirsty as so often is the real issue!

The way you eat will become a habit and if it is not healthy it is time to change the habit. You do not need to change it all at once. For some people, making a drastic change can be a little too much and then they fall off the wagon. It is better to change a little bit of behaviour at a time, which is easier to manage, and then you can stay on the right track until you complete all the changes necessary. Obviously the more unhealthy habits you can change the greater the benefit, but pace yourself. Draw up a list of the habits you would like to change and then prioritise them. Start with the ones you have listed as the most important, like cutting back on your sugar consumption, or opting to have a protein breakfast rather than the usual sugar laden cereal, or eating more slowly. Bring in a change a week, or every two weeks. Just think by doing it this way, within a few months you will be eating completely differently and it will be your knew habit. Slowly, slowly, catch that monkey!

You will not feel the difference immediately, although I have known many people to feel different within three days to a week. Patience is a must, with yourself, and the outcome. And the journey is every bit as important as the end result, to be savoured and enjoyed along the way. Anything you do to promote your own good health is well worth the personal effort. Forget the quick fix, it does not exist my friend......never has, and maybe never will. Time and effort will bring the rewards your way!

A great way to start any new, healthy regime, would be to clean your body of all the mess and junk you have accumulated over the years. Just as if you would spring clean your home, a detox, which need not mean drinking green juice and starving yourself, is always a great start. The major organs involved in elimination are the intestines, the liver, the lungs, the kidneys, and the skin. By detoxing you will aid all these organs in the work they do to keep you fit and healthy. It's equivalent to the pre-wash on your washing machine! With any kind of health kick, from adjusting your weight, to balancing your thyroid, lowering your blood pressure or getting fit, it all works much better if your body is working as effectively as possible before you begin. When your metabolism is boosted and your liver and kidneys are functioning smoothly, it is easier for your body to burn fat, use its nutrients effectively, clear toxins and waste from your organs and deliver the results you want to see. It's a bit like de-scaling your kettle –it will work more efficiently and cost effectively after being cleaned, giving you cleaner clearer water at the end of the boil.

Detoxing doesn't have to be confined to what you eat. Perhaps you could spend a little time detoxing your mind from any negative build up. Clear it of any junk that you do not need to store .Detox your life too. Get rid of anything and/or anybody you do not need anymore, from the pile of newspapers on the desk, to that friend who drains you of your energy.

I will give you now a very simple five day detox to

follow. It is uncomplicated and easy to do and still involves the pleasure of eating, although it will consist of only 'clean' foods. If I have not included a food, then it's not in the five day detox, so there is no need to ask, 'can I have......?'. I have written down all that you can eat, so draw up a lovely list of these things and feel free to eat as much of them as you want. If you can, go organic with the produce to limit chemical intake. Ensure you drink at least 1.5 litres of water every day.

Easy five day detox

Day one: Eat only apples, in any way you like, raw, stewed or baked. Drink fresh apple juice or water and nothing else today. That's it and this is the hardest day, but you will find as you get going you will not mind at all (Anyone with serious health issues or who are pregnant are **not** advised to follow an apple diet. If in doubt please consult with your health care professional).

Day two and three: Have an apple, and include any vegetables you like and any other fruit too. Be inventive with stir fries, soups, roasted vegetables and salads. You can use olive oil and cider vinegar as a dressing. For day two and three you can also drink herbal/fruit teas as well as water.

Day four: Continue to eat and drink as per day two and three and also include brown rice or quinoa.

Day five: Eat and drink as per day four and include either two eggs, a piece of chicken or some fish.

Very simple, yes? And done and dusted in five days! You will probably drop a kilo or two and feel quite high by the end! On the downside, you may struggle around day three, only because you will be eating 'clean' food and no junk at all. You may feel lethargic, you may have headaches and you may feel like you have the flu...or you may not....it all depends on how much your body has to dump in the detox bin! Just remember when you are feeling 'off', your body is doing well and doing its job and once you get over the bad day, you will fly and probably feel euphoric! If you are a real caffeine or sugar addict, just do one day of detox a week for about a month, to gently ease you in – going cold turkey is not always the best route. And cut down on the amount of caffeine and/or sugar you consume each week. Ask your doctor if you are concerned or if you have major health issues.

After your gentle detox, on which you can spend any amount of time, it need not be just five days, it could be, like I say, just one day to a few weeks- it is time to focus on your diet. The problem with many weight loss plans or lifestyle diet changes is they focus on the foods you cannot eat. By doing this the diet is a negative process from the very beginning where the brain is fed thoughts of deprivation. It is far more beneficial to focus on what you can have, drawing up lists of all the incredible foods that will bring your body into balance and have you jumping out of bed with boundless energy and enthusiasm for life. That is how I work, this is what brings my client's incredible results, this is how you can get the beautiful fit and healthy body you so deserve. This is the positive attitude towards our food that we need.

I want to make this new way of eating really easy and uncomplicated for you, so it is a doddle to follow and implement into your daily life. So here goes:

Forget everything that is processed, made from white flour, marketed as a fast food (whether it be a cereal bar, take-away or a microwave meal) and anything you **KNOW** is not a healthy choice. Just remove it all from your brain, your cupboards and your shopping list my friend. Act like all that stuff does not and never has existed. Now draw your focus, your thoughts and your energies to all that is great in the world of food! Let the feast begin......

Fruit and vegetables

I am sure you have heard about eating your five a day, but five portions of fruit or vegetables a day is really a minimum rather than a maximum. In reality you need to aim for eight a day as your optimum intake. Due to sugar content, you will be better off increasing your vegetable intake rather than the amount of fruit you eat. Variety, as they say, is the spice of life, and this is certainly so when it comes to the variety of vegetables and fruit you should consume. The greater the variety, the higher your chances are of receiving the vast array of different nutrients you require to dance in the rain! If you are like me, and cannot digest fruit well (and do not particularly enjoy it), aim for more vegetables. If you are not particularly fond of vegetables, do your best to disguise them in soups, which is an easy way to get your hit.

A favourite salad of mine is sliced fresh beetroot, and sliced beef tomato, topped with a clove or two of crushed garlic, olive oil and feta cheese.

Vegetables can be raw, cooked, fresh, or frozen (frozen vegetables are often more fresh than those on the supermarket shelves as they are frozen on the day they are harvested). Do your best to have some raw vegetables every day. Raw vegetables have the greatest chance of being nutrient and enzyme rich as you haven't cooked the life, and the goodness, out of them. Be inventive with salads and eat crudité's as a snack. Steam your vegetables or stir fry them my friend, in order to retain greater nutrition –an added bonus is that this method of cooking is also quick and easy.

Here is a perfect munch that keeps the calories low and the nutrients high – dip radishes into hummus. Radishes have less than 1 calorie each and are 95%% water so they keep you hydrated too! Humus contains protein, so combined they should keep you going for longer as well as nourishing your body.

One portion of green vegetables is either two spears of broccoli or a couple of heaped tablespoons of kale, spinach or green beans. A portion of carrots, peas or sweetcorn is equivalent to a couple of heaped tablespoons and a portion of salad is three sticks of celery, a 5cm piece of cucumber or a few cherry tomatoes. You see it is not that difficult to get your eight a day, and if you have a great salad, or a bowl of homemade vegetable soup, you are already well on your way. Top that off with a snack or two of fruit and you will be hitting the jackpot!

Make fruit your daily treat instead of the crisps, sweets, or a sugary bun! Turn bananas or a few strawberries into a delicious indulgence by dipping them in a few squares of melted dark chocolate. Try to eat fruit alone and not with your main meals as fruit digests very quickly and can sit and ferment whilst waiting for you to finish digesting fats and protein. Melon, which is often served as an after dinner snack, is one of the worse fruits to eat with any other food as melon gets digested more quickly than anything else. Many people suffer from digestive problems when they finish their meal off with a bowl of fresh fruit salad, or a pile of grapes and would never think to blame the healthy fruit! On the other hand an apple with a handful of nuts, or a small piece of cheese, makes for a perfectly well- balanced snack.

Fruit is also a great way to begin your day and made into a smoothie with a small amount of protein such as natural, 'live' yogurt, or some ground almonds, will set your digestion and energy on the right path for a super charged day.

Just as with vegetables, eat fruit that is in season and not fruit that is produced all year round by synthetic growing means. Fruits grown by these methods may have depleted nutrient value, less fibre and more sugar – which, as you know, can make you pile on the pounds! Worse still it can play with your insulin levels which lead to Metabolic Syndrome and Diabetes type 2. Sorry to harp on about it but organic will be best again, saving you from the chemical treatments and giving you fruit much higher in antioxidants – you know, those nutrients that help to prevent you developing disease such as cancer.

A delicious Chocolate and Pear Smoothie

- *1 Banana*
- *1 Pear*
- *500ml of a milk alternative, such as almond, quinoa or rice milk or use some goat/sheep yogurt and a little water*
- *I teaspoon of raw cocoa powder and some ground nuts of your choice, such as ground almonds or hazelnuts*

Put all the ingredients in a blender and whiz away. Makes for a healthy way to begin your day, a sweet treat when you need one, or acts as a fab post work out snack.
If you like avocado you could use half an avocado instead of the pear which will bring its own unique spectrum of nutrition. When you have peeled your half avocado to use in the smoothie, don't waste the other half. Squeeze lemon juice onto the unpeeled half and place in the fridge for later. Use the flesh side of the peeled skin, as a face wipe and natural face pack. Once you have wiped the skin over your face, you will look like a little green Martian, but leave it on for five minutes and then rinse off. You will have radiant, soft, nourished skin!

One portion of fruit is either two small fruits such as plums, apricot, or satsumas; one medium fruit such as an apple, pear or orange; or half a large fruit such as grapefruit or a large slice of pineapple or mango. One serving of dried fruit is about 30g.

Paint a rainbow in your mind and find a fruit or vegetable to fit every colour. Do your best to eat different coloured fruit and vegetables each day, but not in a huge variety at each meal time. Remember we would probably only have eaten one kind of fruit and vegetable at each meal thousands of years ago, and we need to remain fairly simple to optimise digestion. Do some research on the internet or in books for coloured fruits and vegetables and compile your own colour chart of these life enhancing super foods, you will be sure to discover a few you have forgotten about!

If you are trying to convince your little ones to eat their fruit and vegetables decorate their plates with them in various fun ways. Again, just by doing a little bit of research you will find all kinds of weird and wonderful ways to turn fruit and vegetables into colourful characters and scenes, from palm trees on beaches to Halloween characters. If you really have trouble getting your little ones to eat their 8 a day, disguise them in soups, mashed potato, homemade pasta sauces and even homemade ice lollies!

Make fruit and vegetables something to look forward to, exciting and appealing. Cook them lightly, savour the crunch as you eat them and burn extra calories as you do.! My friend, your vegetables long to be the main focus on your plate, with the largest space dedicated to them in honour of their glorious life giving properties. Indulge and enjoy.

Protein – meat, fish, eggs, nuts, seeds, dairy and legumes

Protein is vital for growth, repair of tissues, enzymes, hormones, neurotransmitters, and forms approximately 22% of your body (second only to water). It needs to be replenished each day. Protein is found in meat, fish, nuts, seeds, eggs, cheese, milk, beans and pulses, but, as with everything you eat, it is the quality of the protein that counts. It has been shown, and you are welcome to research this for yourself, that people who eat a diet high in meat and dairy have a much lower health rating. There is a direct link to heart disease and cancer,

---

Easy, peasey Chicken Risotto

It can be very time consuming to make a real risotto but here is a cheat's version. I am all for healthy food that is quick and easy!

- *1 onion, chopped*
- *1or 2 crushed garlic cloves to suit your taste*
- *1 small tin of sweetcorn, a few sliced mushrooms slices of red/yellow/green pepper*
- *1 chicken breast diced (you can add more if you are cooking for more than 1 or 2 people)*
- *Slightly undercooked brown basmati rice (225g/8 oz before cooking)*
- *240ml/8fl oz stock, a large handful of chopped fresh coriander (you could use a couple of teaspoons of dried coriander if you wish)*
- *A glass of white wine (for the risotto you understand!).*

Gently fry the onion and garlic in some olive/coconut oil until the onion just starts to soften.
Add the chicken and continue to cook for approximately 5 minutes, then add the mushrooms and pepper slices and allow them to soften.
Add the rest of the ingredients and bring to the boil. Simmer, stirring occasionally, until everything is well cooked and most of the stock has been absorbed. Season with salt and pepper.

---

particularly colon cancer in meat eaters and hormonal cancers such as breast and prostate for dairy consumers. Really neither meat nor milk should be a seven day a week staple of your diet, and the best diets include a couple of meat free days a week. Give your digestive system and your body as a whole, a day or two without meat to recover, rejuvenate, and rejoice! Seriously, your body will thank you for it.

Eat lean meat if you are a meat eater, with the emphasis more on white meat than red meat. Invest those few extra pennies (or pounds) where you can and opt for organic, which will have a smaller content of hormones and antibiotics (you do not need these added extras interfering with your body). I understand that organic meat, or any other produce for that matter, can be more expensive, but if you find the balance and eat less, making it go further, the cost will be equal to eating a larger amount of poor quality meat. (The investment will far out -weigh the disease promoting qualities of cheaper, non-organic meat.)

Another great source of protein is fish and seafood. Seafood/fish is considered to be a low calorie food when compared to other protein-rich foods such as meat and poultry. Most lean or lower fat species of fish, such as cod and sole, contain 100 calories or less per 3 ounce cooked portion, and even the fattier fish like mackerel, herring, and salmon contain approximately 200 calories or less in a 3 ounce cooked serving. It is a high quality protein with all the essential amino acids required for good health. Fish is easier to digest than meat because it has less connective tissue, making it a better choice for those with digestive issues, those who have been sick and/ or the elderly for example.

Baked Trout with Lemon and herbs

I love easy fish meals like this one. You could substitute other herbs for the parsley in this recipe such as coriander, basil, tarragon or a mixture of more than one. And you could use a different fish if you do not like Trout, for example salmon fillets, or a fillet of cod.

- *1 rainbow trout*
- *a handful of chopped fresh parsley (or other herbs)*
- *½ level tsp mustard*
- *the juice of a lemon and some butter to spread on the fish*

Set the oven temperature to 180 degrees. Place the fish in the centre of a piece of foil and spread the top with butter and place a small knob of butter inside the fish.
Mix the chopped parsley with the mustard and lemon juice. Spread this mixture on top of the fish and place a little inside. Wrap the foil around the fish to make a parcel and place in the oven for approximately 25 minutes. Serve with a side salad or some stir fry vegetables. Delicious and easy!

Eat fish three times a week, or up to five times. Again though, be aware of the quality and go for wild or sea- reared fish rather than farmed. Oily fish such as tuna, mackerel, sardines and salmon also offer a fabulous dose of essential fats that you need to include in your diet. Prawns are even lower in calories and fat than chicken yet have much more protein. As well as being high in protein, prawns contain Omega 3 fats, magnesium, iron, zinc and magnesium. Grilled, oven baked, stir fried – these are just some of the ways to cook your fish. You can even throw it on the BBQ, during those beautiful warm, sunny days, just ensure you cook it thoroughly, but never burn it.

Eggs are a perfect way to start your day and are a great source of protein. Eggs give us numerous vitamins, including vitamin A, potassium and many B vitamins like folic acid, choline and biotin and they are one of the rare sources of vitamin D. Yes they do contain cholesterol, but we need a certain amount of beneficial cholesterol, which eggs contain. I remember when I was very sick all those years ago, my nutritionist insisted that I started every single day with an egg to bring me back from the dead and to kick start my energy in the morning. I was not a huge fan of eggs, (or breakfast!) but it worked. Trust me; an egg is a far superior way to start your day than the bowl of sugar laden cereal. Eat them in moderation, of course, but do get your eggs in and it goes without saying, that free range are the better option, both for you and the chickens!

Here is a delicious, simple and nutritious meal idea for any time of the day and a favourite quick meal of mine and my eldest son: Make scrambled eggs, but mix in feta cheese, tuna, sliced tomato and a teaspoon of turmeric. A wonderful protein hit that will keep you going for hours!

Nuts and seeds are a great source of protein and are extremely nutrient-dense. Along with protein, they provide generous amounts of healthy fats, complex carbohydrates, vitamins, minerals and fibre. Trace minerals like magnesium, zinc, selenium and copper are important but may be under-consumed in today's' largely processed' Western diet, and this may even still be the case in some plant-based diets. Nuts and seeds are a reliable and delicious source of these essential nutrients. The good news is that eating the right portion of nuts and seeds (about one handful each day) can help you lose or maintain weight by satiating your appetite, but it is important not to eat too many as they are very high in calories! So don't sit there and eat the whole bag (not something I would ever do, of course) stick to the handful a day. They can also stabilize your blood-sugar levels and improve your cholesterol and triglycerides, which may reduce your risk of type 2 diabetes and heart disease. Nutty not to indulge!

The king of nuts is the Macadamia .It contains all the essential amino acids, various forms of fibre, and high levels of vitamins and minerals. Its fat content is predominantly monounsaturated fat so helps to raise HDL (good cholesterol) and lower LDL (bad cholesterol). Macadamia nuts are rich and satisfying, making them a superb snack. Keep a few in your bag for those times when hunger attacks – better than reaching for the crisps or sweet snacks.

Quinoa, which we use like a grain, is a complete protein, and has all 9 essential amino acids which is, great for a vegetarian diet. It is very high in manganese that helps keep bones strong and healthy and maintain normal blood sugar levels. It is high in fibre and contains niacin, both of which have been demonstrated to lower and control high cholesterol.. It is easy to prepare, and can be used in any recipe or meal that calls for rice. It is naturally gluten-free and also makes perfect sweets and porridge.

Pre prepared Quinoa lunches.

Prepare this simple recipe and use over a few days as packed lunches for work (or school).
Wash some quinoa (amount depending on how much you wish to make) and then fry for a couple of minutes with an onion and some garlic (if you like it).
Add water (it will give you the amounts on the quinoa pack) and simmer for 15 – 20 minutes.
When it is finished take off the heat and add: Tuna or cooked, diced chicken, sweetcorn, diced peppers, fresh chopped tomatoes (a tin of chopped tomatoes if you prefer life to be more easy), some herbs of your choice, fresh or dried,, salt and pepper to taste. This also makes a quick and delicious family meal!

Dairy is a source of protein, calcium and vitamin D and does offer some health benefits this way. Just keep your dairy products to a minimum – you have already read my concerns! Use cheese as a snack with an apple, or have some natural, 'live' yogurt (which also contains friendly bacteria and live enzymes for digestion) with berries, walnuts and a drizzle of local honey for breakfast. If you like a spread on your bread, make it butter, as at least butter is a source of vitamin A and E and healthy saturated fats, and not margarine as margarine is another unhealthy commodity full of highly processed trans fats which are toxic! (Better still use health promoting nut butters such as almond or walnut butter – yummy!)

Beans and pulses are known as the poor man's protein. They are cheap to eat, yet have the added benefit of being virtually fat free and cholesterol free – unlike their animal equivalent. I am sure here is something you did not know - beans and pulses also count as one of your 5(8) a day, which include any beans, chickpeas and lentils. One portion is three heaped tablespoons but no matter how much you eat in a day it will still count as one portion towards your 5(8) a day. It is also best you do not go over this amount as they tend to cause

Bean Bolognese

This is a great for one of your meat free days!

- *1 tablespoon olive oil*
- *1 onion chopped*
- *2 cloves garlic crushed*
- *1 tsp mixed herbs*
- *some mushrooms*
- *4 beef tomatoes chopped*
- *1 stock cube*
- *1 tablespoon tomato puree*
- *1 can of beans such as Borlotti, Cannellini or pinto beans, drained and rinsed*

Sauté the onion, garlic and herbs for 2 minutes, add the mushrooms and tomatoes and cook until soft. Add the stock cube, tomato puree and beans. Season and simmer for 10 minutes.
Serve with brown basmati rice, wholegrain pasta or as a filling for a jacket potato!
You can make this up in advance and freeze it in individual portions for a quick, healthy meal later in the week.

wind in the digestive tract that can be somewhat uncomfortable and embarrassing if you are not in the company of people who have a childish sense of humour! Added to your homemade soup, where they can be disguised, or made into salads, you top up your 5 a day and get a great, cholesterol free, inexpensive, portion of protein. Way to go!

Begin your day with some quality, lean protein, be it a little live yogurt topped with some walnuts, or some smoked salmon, an egg or some beans. You should eat a small amount of protein at every mealtime my friend, as protein will keep you feeling fuller for longer and will give you energy and muscle building power. When you eat protein you will also supply other nutrients for your body such as the B vitamin group, iron, magnesium, zinc and essential fats. We were designed to run on protein, and being as we are 22% protein, it is good and healthy to keep our levels topped up!

The Essential Fats

Any nutrient named as essential is a substance the body must have in order to survive. The body cannot manufacture essential nutrients and so it is necessary to get them from our diet. If the body obtains too little of an essential nutrient, ill health will follow, and may be even death.

Over time fats have been subject to much criticism with reference to health and weight issues, most notably with the promotion of fat free diets, leading people to do their best to avoid fat at all costs. However, ironically, a diet without fat has been shown to cause health and weight issues! Fat deficiency symptoms include: weakness, fatigue, high blood pressure, inflammation in tissues, weak eyesight, depression, impaired cognitive function, hair loss, slow wound healing, miscarriage in females, water retention, hyperactivity, elevated cholesterol and weight gain. There are many more symptoms, but I think you get the general idea.

> Take a basic salad of green leaves (such as spinach, watercress and Cos lettuce) and add to it some lean protein such as fish, chicken, turkey or cooked lentils for protein replenishment, slices of avocado for healthy essential fatty acids and Vitamin E for immune support, plus brown rice or quinoa for fibre and minerals. Top it off with some sliced tomato which contains the compound Lycopene, which speeds up muscle recovery after exercise and helps lower blood glucose levels. Use a drizzle of olive oil for appetite control and a sprinkle of mixed dried herbs and flax seeds for extra taste. Super eating! Super tasty!

We need fats and the two essential fatty acids are known as Omega 3 and Omega 6. The best supplies of the essential Omegas are mackerel, herring, tuna, salmon, anchovies, haddock, trout and sardines. Good vegetarian sources are flax seeds, flaxseed oil, rapeseed oil, hemp oil and walnuts. All green leafy vegetables contain a precursor of Omega 3. Spinach, seaweeds and spirulina are also great sources of Omega 3. Wild game is rich in Omega 3 as it feeds on grass and not grain. Eggs from free range chickens can provide up to twenty times more Omega 3 than grain fed chicken eggs. And avocados are a rich source too. So there is plenty of great food out there to get your essential supply.

Grains

A dietary staple for some 10,000 years, grains are the seeds of cereal crops and include wheat, rye, rice, millet, oats, maize and barley as well as some less common kinds. However grains can cause digestive upset, as 10,000 years in evolutionary terms is not a long time for us to have evolved to be able to digest them. If you suffer from indigestion following eating products that contain grains, it is a clear indication that you are having problems digesting. If you suffer any digestive problems, a grain free diet may help. Pin point what is causing your problem and do your best to eliminate it.

A bowl of porridge oats for breakfast (the only cereal I promote) or as a snack in the day will help soothe stomach discomfort as well as being a good source of fibre and energy. Sprinkle with a little cinnamon to help lower blood sugar levels. Top it with some crushed walnuts for heart health, a drizzle of honey for immune protection and a little seasonal fruit for extra vitamins and minerals.

There is clear scientific evidence supporting the role of grains, especially whole-grains, in the reduced risk of chronic diseases such as heart disease, type 2 diabetes and cancer. But the message is clear and simple my friend - 'Go brown and whole'. Enjoy your wholemeal bread, and baking with brown flours. Use brown basmati rice to accompany your meals and

Gluten Free Pitta Breads

The biggest complaint of being Gluten free is finding decent bread that does not taste like hardboard, and is also of a reasonable price! If you are a fellow gluten free buddy, or you fancy going gluten free to help with digestive complaints, here is a quick and simple recipe for making some delicious pitta breads. You can also use this recipe for a fantastic, light and fluffy pizza base. As an added bonus, there is no yeast, no sugar and no added salt! Perfect for those on a yeast free/sugar free diet and a much healthier option to some breads!

- 200g natural yogurt
- 200g gluten free flour
- 1 egg and....that's it! (Yep, that's it! Uncomplicated my friend, as always!)

Mix the ingredients together in a bowl and then divide the dough into five or six balls.

Place the balls on a well- floured baking sheet and then flatten the balls with your hands (great for a bit of stress busting) shaping into nice round pita breads.

Bake for approx. 15 minutes at 190 degrees. Simple!

If you want to make a pizza base from this instead of pitta breads, after making the dough do not divide into balls, but press out the dough into a pizza base on the baking sheet. Add your toppings and then bake for about 20 minutes at 190 degrees.

You could also make it into large garlic bread, or make very little balls to make garlic balls.

I have even found that this mix makes a good substitute pastry and have made delicious quiches with it! The only issue with the mix is that it does not roll out well with a rolling pin. You need to flatten it by pressing it with your hands – more floury fun!

drizzle it with quality Olive or avocado oil for extra taste and nutrients.

Apart from the health benefits already mentioned, quinoa, which we use like a grain, happens to have a low glycaemic index compared to other whole grains. The glycaemic index – or GI – rates food based on how much they make your blood sugar rise. Keeping your blood sugar steady and balanced can help you to maintain a balanced weight, reduce cholesterol levels and help with many other health issues– that's why whole unprocessed foods that are low in sugar and high in fibre (like whole grains) are touted for their health benefits.

Water

The best drink you can have is, no not coffee or beer, water! We are predominately made up of water, in fact we are one giant walking puddle, and so need to keep our water levels topped up so that we do not become dehydrated and dry out like a prune! Water is the most abundant substance in our body, found in virtually every part of us except bone and tooth enamel! It stabilizes our temperature, dissolves reactants so that reactions may occur in our body, helps the intestines eliminate waste and absorb nutrients and also flushes toxins and waste materials out.

Most of us do not drink anywhere near enough water and tend to blame everything else for our ills, rather than acknowledging that a lot of our problems could be down to having a lack of water in the body. Your skin can be a great sign of dehydration. If you have very dry skin or you are looking more wrinkled than you should, trust me, you need to drink more water. A headache can be a good sign that you need hydrating, so before you go grabbing the painkillers, sip some water for half an hour and see if the headache goes - after all better water in your system than pharmaceutical drugs!

Green tea with mint and lime is great for fat burning, digestion, headaches, congestion and breath freshness.

I know water can be very boring to drink, but liven it up with slices of lemon, lime, orange or ginger. Add mint and slices of cucumber, or cinnamon. Use naturally carbonated spring water for something with a little sparkle. Have a cup of hot water with slices of ginger in and sip it to help to control acid reflux. By adding some mint leaves you will also help to flush the acid from your system! By starting your day with a glass of hot water with slices of lemon you will detox your system and spark your metabolism. Plus packed full of vitamin C, the lemon will give your immune system an instant boost!

Because of the amount of chemicals used in drinking water, it is probably healthier to consume filtered water.

Drink a glass of water as soon as you wake up and another before you go to bed and sip some throughout the day. When I say sip, I do mean sip. If you gulp down the water you will only flood your system and your body will expel it quickly to regain the balance and so a lot will be not used to any benefit.

Your tea and coffee, which have their own health benefits, do form part of your daily water consumption, as do your fruit and vegetables, but there is nothing better for you than plain, unadulterated water.

Set yourself the challenge of drinking 1.5 litres a day. Measure the amount out and then ensure you sip away throughout the day. If you find this a lot to get through, you are probably not drinking enough on a daily basis. Aim for 1.5 litres a day as a minimum and see the difference in your health and energy.

Herbs and Spices

Herbs and spices are not mentioned in many diet books and they are not usually on the list of a balanced diet. However, they have such great health properties, and add awesome flavour to food that I believe they are worth a mention and should be added to your daily intake. Use them in your everyday cooking so that you do not miss the unhealthy added fats, sugar and salt. Here are a few examples:

Turmeric is a bright yellow spice which contains the active compound curcumin. Curcumin has a variety of powerful anti-inflammatory actions without the side effects that prescription drugs have. There are further research studies on the potential role of turmeric in preventing acute respiratory distress syndrome, liver cancer, and post-menopausal osteoporosis. It has great antibiotic and antiseptic properties and can be used in the treatment of cuts and burns. Great to use whilst indulging in a detox as it detoxes the liver. The Chinese have used it for many years to help treat depression and research on mice has shown the slowing of multiple sclerosis. With all those fabulous health benefits, and many more that I have not mentioned I recommend that you get a teaspoon a day, where you can, into your diet. Delicious when you add it to curries, soups and scrambled eggs and you could even add some to your morning smoothie.

> I have a client with Multiple Sclerosis who takes a supplement of turmeric and ginger every day to keep inflammation under control. I have several clients with digestive issues, from Crohn's to diverticulitis who use a liquid supplement that includes turmeric to keep gut inflammation down and another client who uses turmeric in her cooking every day, and I mean every day, to keep her arthritis at bay! I use turmeric to clean my teeth as it keeps them white!

Rosemary not only tastes good in dishes with chicken, lamb, and roasted vegetables, but it is also a good source of iron, calcium, and vitamin B6. Rosemary was traditionally used to help alleviate muscle pain, improve memory, boost the immune and circulatory system, and promote hair growth. Now there is growing evidence of the role Rosemary plays as a potent anti -cancer compound, with promising results in studies of its efficacy against breast cancer, prostate cancer, colon cancer, leukaemia, and skin cancer. It boosts immunity, circulation, mood and memory, aids digestive upset, relieves water retention, and freshens breath. If you drink rosemary wine it is said to improve appetite and improve digestion....

sounds like a plan to me!

Oregano, (of which I am particularly fond, especially when sprinkled over my salads) has a substantial number of health claims associated with its potent antioxidants and anti-bacterial properties. The herb is used to treat respiratory tract disorders, gastrointestinal (GI) disorders, menstrual cramps, and urinary tract disorders. Not bad eh? It contains fibre, iron, manganese, vitamin E, iron, calcium, omega fatty acids, manganese, and tryptophan, plus Vitamin K - an important vitamin which promotes bone growth, the maintenance of bone density, and the production of blood clotting proteins. Wow, that was a long list in a short breath! Add it to your oils for salads, dash it over your tomatoes, sprinkle on your homemade pizza, in your homemade tomato sauces, vegetarian dishes and meat dishes as well, for example, your homemade meatballs and let the beautiful aroma lift your senses.

The spice cumin originated in the Mediterranean, and it was used extensively by the Greeks, the Romans, the Egyptians, the Persians, and just about everyone else in that region! It appears to provide a number of potential health benefits, these include acting as an anti-glycation agent, antioxidant and anti-osteoporotic. It is very beneficial for digestion as the seeds help in the secretion of pancreatic enzymes that aids in proper digestion and helps in absorption of the nutrients. It is rich in Vitamin E, which helps keep the skin remain healthy and young and free from fungal and bacterial infection. It has been shown to reduce stress and insomnia, so a great spice my friend, to flavour your supper! It is fabulous in curries, soups or just about any other dish you want to aromatically spice up. I love mixing it with garlic, orange juice, lemon juice and a little olive oil to baste fish. Mix cumin with tahini, garlic and olive oil, and stir into a green salad for a lightly spiced dressing.

Mint is one of the oldest and most popular herbs that has been grown around the world. It soothes the digestive tract and if you are having stomach ache then it can be of great help. It also cleanses the stomach, clears up skin disorders, eliminates toxins, freshens your breath and cleanses the blood. Fabulous as a tea, or served fresh over ice with sparkling water for a cool summer drink. (Add a slice of lemon and cucumber to have a superb detox drink, also particularly lovely in the summer.) Mix mint with live yogurt for a delicious dip that is also beneficial for digestive discomfort.

Improve the flavour of your homemade tomato soup and at the same time improve your cardiovascular health by adding basil. With both anti- bacterial and anti- inflammatory properties basil is an excellent source of vitamin K and a very good source of iron, calcium and vitamin A. In addition, basil is a good source of dietary fibre, manganese, magnesium, vitamin C and potassium. Enjoy a taste of Italy by layering fresh basil leaves over slices of tomato and mozzarella cheese to create this traditional, colourful and delicious salad and you could even add a few slices of avocado to give an even greater nutrient kick. Delicious! Grow it on your window sills to keep mosquitoes away and to be able to enjoy the soothing aroma.

If you like it hot, fire up the chillies. The main component in chillies is a chemical called Capsaicin, which is responsible for the intense heat felt, but what else does the red hot chilli pepper do? If you eat it with your meal it helps to control insulin release and thus controls blood sugars and helps in the maintenance of weight. Chillies improve the health of your heart, boost circulation, thin the blood, help protect against strokes, reduces inflammation, helps aid relaxation and are great for pain relief. Chillies have been shown to stop the spread of prostate cancer and lower the risk of colon cancer. Have there ever been greater reasons to spice up your life?

Chickpea lunch

Here's a very quick and healthy lunch.
- *1 tin of chickpeas, drained*
- *1 teaspoon cumin*
- *1 teaspoon Paprika*
- *1 tablespoon Tahini*
- *1 teaspoon olive oil*
- *(Optional) I tablespoon natural live yogurt*

Heat the chickpeas in a pan with all the other ingredients (except the yogurt, if you are using it, which you add after you have heated the chickpeas), then serve with some home- made crusty wholemeal bread or some gluten free pitta bread.

Cinnamon adds wonderful flavour to homemade cakes, especially those with mixed dried fruit. When I use cinnamon, I find that any form of sugar used in the baking can be greatly reduced. Cinnamon is believed to control blood sugar levels and as so, is great for those with diabetes, hyperglycaemia and those wanting to have constant energy and a good mood. It has been found to be effective for helping with premenstrual pain, and for lowering cholesterol. It contains fibre, calcium, iron, and manganese, so sprinkle it on your morning porridge, in your smoothies, or on your cappuccino (if you are still indulging in milk!). Make a delicious dessert of baked apples sprinkled with cinnamon, or stew some apple with cinnamon and eat with live, natural yogurt. If you have a cold, drink hot water with lemon, cinnamon and a drizzle of honey. Cinnamon's oils and nutrient composition can reduce the symptoms of the virus. Of course cinnamon can be used in savoury dishes too, giving them a rather exotic taste.

Not only do herbs and spices add flavour to your food my friend, they also offer amazing health benefits. You do not need unhealthy fats, salt and sugar when adding natural flavour from nature's own spice rack and medicine cupboard to your cooking. Do some research into herbs and spices yourself, there is plenty of information out there both on the net and in books.

Summary for a balanced diet

The foundations of a balanced diet, for the average person (not that we are ever average) - and this is not taking into account if you are vegetarian, have food allergies, or any other particular health issues/ lifestyle needs - should contain a range of fruit and vegetables, nuts, seeds, beans, lentils, quality meat and fish, and whole grains; with a nibble of dairy, a sprinkle of herbs and spices and plenty of water. Uncomplicated and simple really wouldn't you agree? No need to make it any more difficult than that. Keep it simple my friend.

If you think about it, this is the diet that nature provides, the diet that nature intended for us. These foods - untouched by the processing industry which destroys nutrients and adds harmful ingredients such as chemicals and excess salts and sugars - are enough to keep us fit and well. By eating such a diet you will be using a form of preventative medicine that will keep you protected from disease and bouncing with energy for life!

A person's diet is an individual matter and you are the best judge of what is right for you, but if you need professional help, as we all do from time to time, seek it. Discover the best diet for you. Remember you are as unique as your DNA and your diet should be tailored for the individual you are. Once you are on the right diet, your body will thank you for it, and you should be able to reap the benefits of fabulous health. Just by keeping to what nature has provided for you, you will be on the right path!

Let's just finish this section on a light note my friend. I am a great believer in a little of what you fancy does you good, and if you occasionally have some food that is not on the healthy list, providing it is not a daily occurrence, of course, it's perfectly okay to do so! Fine dark chocolate, red wine and champagne are my luscious indulgences - enjoyed without reproach! You too should have, and enjoy, your indulgences.

Learn to love the food you eat and learn to eat the food that loves you in return.

Exercise - Moderation is key
- bet that pleased you and I aim to please!

"My grandmother started walking five miles a day when she
was sixty. She's ninety-seven now, and we don't know where
the heck she is."
— Ellen DeGeneres

If you take care of your body my friend, your body will
take care of you. Exercise and good nutrition are the foundations
of great health. Regular, moderate exercise can ease depression
and anxiety, boost energy and mood, trim your waistline,
improve your sex life, and relieve stress. No matter what your
age or fitness level, exercise will have plenty of positive benefits
for you. It is a perfect way to feel fantastic and have a vibrant
feeling of well- being.

So, with all the fabulous benefits on offer, why is it
the word 'exercise' is like swearing for some people? In my
practising experience, there are more people who dislike the
idea of exercise than those who love it and there are far more
people who abstain from exercise than there are those who
partake in it. Yet, as I have said there are so many health
benefits to be gained from exercise and just to expand on what
I have already said - exercise can help you feel more energetic
throughout the day, it can aid a better night's sleep, give you
a sharper memory, and help you relax. Of course exercise can
make vast improvements to your physique too so it does seem

a wee bit of a shame to miss out!

For the most part those who say they do not like exercising actually mean they do not like the form of exercise they have in mind. I have to say that if exercise meant running 5km every day for me, I too would be less than keen. I have never run more than 5km and have no intention of doing so. It really is uninspiring for me and not something I would be motivated to do. But put on some music and I will be the Dancing Queen….. All Night Long!

In my consulting experience there seems to be four main reasons people do not engage in exercise (even if you can come up with four hundred!) but I am not going to include the 'I am allergic to exercise' reason here (that's a classic!) :

1.   The gym.

When you mention the word exercise there are those who immediately conjure up the picture of being clad in Lycra, sweating buckets in a testosterone filled gymnasium and feeling sick and miserable as they pound the treadmill. But my friend, it does not have to mean that at all…..not one bit. Unless of course this is the kind of exercise you enjoy and feel motivated to do, in which case, keep banging that treadmill!

2.   Motivation and inspiration

I believe the second main reason people do not exercise is motivation and inspiration or lack of it. Despite all the life-changing benefits, many of us still think of exercise as a chore, suitable only for the young or the athletic. We lack motivation but have plenty of excuses – such as the 'I am allergic to exercise!' Seriously do these people believe that I will empathise with an allergy to exercise?

But back to motivation and inspiration- take as an example the hundreds of New Year resolutions to get fit. The 2nd of January (not the 1st because of the hang over) everyone starts off bright and breezy and determined to improve themselves and the gym memberships are up by at least 30%, much to the delight of the gyms. However for the majority of people the good intentions are short lived –after two months many have lost the motivation, for others two weeks or for the very faint-hearted, just a few days. Why? It's those cold dark nights, the warm winter food, the cosy fireside and the urge to snuggle up under a blanket watching TV after a long day at work which is inspiring. So there is a real lack of inspiration to go and exercise. The comfort zone has far more pull to it than the thought of exercise. Add to that a form of exercise that is not enjoyable and motivation is locked out in the cold too! You need the right motivation and inspiration to keep you going, no matter what the weather, no matter what excuses you want to use.

3.   The financial cost.

It's those awful gym fees, joining fees, and penalties for wanting to quit fees that put people off. It can be an added expense that many cannot afford, or there is always something else each month to spend the money on. However, exercise can be free too! For example, nature has provided us with a marvellous fully equipped, air conditioned, gym just outside our door.

4.   Time.

Everyone is way too busy to find the time to exercise. But there is always time for exercising, when you choose to make it.

You know, my friend, exercise keeps you thinking healthy, which will lead to a host of healthy decisions each day, including what you eat. Then you are set on the road to great health.....which is what this book, and life is all about!

At this point my friend, I hope to change the way you see exercise - to help you understand that exercise merely means moving, raising your heart beat for a few minutes, and challenging your muscles a little. I hope to motivate and inspire you to take a little time out each week to get fit and in so doing, to feel great. I hope to help you understand why exercise is important to your over -all well- being and therefore the quality of your life both now and in the future. There is no reason for you to be a fitness fanatic to reap the benefits nor does it take hours of pumping weights in a gym or running mile after mile to achieve great results. No matter what your age or fitness level, there are lots of enjoyable ways to use physical activity to keep you feeling on top of the world.

What exactly would a simple, moderate exercise program do for you? A ha, sit back and be inspired my friend!

Improve your sense of wellbeing - Yes , forget the X Factor this is the 'feel-good' factor!

Give you a sense of achievement -Each fitness goal you

reach will be like lifting the Trophy!

Clear your thinking and improve your memory - I am sure that would be helpful!?

Improve any anxiety or stress you may be experiencing and elevate your mood – Exercise helps you to feel more relaxed, at ease and lighter in spirits. For example it has been demonstrated to help when treating depression.

Improve your sleep quality - Beautiful restful sleep will bring greater health and it is far more pleasant to have a lovely, peaceful and full night's sleep, than tossing and turning and suffering from insomnia.

Improve your strength, mobility and flexibility – You will be able to get out of bed without feeling stiff, climb the stairs with ease, pick up something from the floor without the need for someone to help you stand up after and have no problem to keep going all day.

Help you reduce the chance of developing chronic health problems such as heart disease and diabetes - Is there a better reason to exercise?

For those with existing heart disease, diabetes or high blood pressure, exercise has the potential to improve how well the condition is controlled and even the possibility of reducing medication!

Help with weight loss and body toning and aid in the maintenance of muscle during weight loss - A way to get that beautiful beach body –remember fit is the new skinny!

Improve your posture, which in turn will aid in the placement and thus the workings of your inner organs - When your posture is bad, your organs can become slightly misplaced, which hinders the body's ability to work effectively.

Put the spark back into your sex life! - Exercise will enhance your performance and staying power so there will be no problem swinging from the chandeliers!

Quite an impressive list, isn't it? And I could have made it longer! I am sure we would all like to feel good every day, to have that 'Feel Good Factor', and so even if we consider just this one point, it makes sense to do at least some exercise.

To better understand what exercise should be comprised of, let's take a moment to understand what our ancestors in their sexy loin clothes would have been up to without the treadmill and bench press! There are five basic movements that we use every day and should use every day: squatting, pushing, pulling, lifting and lunging. Our ancestors would have, for example, squatted to eat and to defecate, lifted heavy things to build shelters or move obstacles from their path (or carried a big kill), they would have pulled up roots , and pushed down trees and they would have used lunges as they climbed hills or fought animals. If they ran, it would have been in short sharp bursts to chase a kill or to not be a meal!. Our ancestors would have walked/wandered around all day (not sat in front of a computer or in a car) in search of food and water so they would have been constantly moving. All this adds up to why they were so very fit, lean and strong. (Plus their great unprocessed diet, of course!)

Our ancestors would not have physically worked out hard for hours, such as a long gym session, or just for an hour, such as the average gym session, and then have sat around for the rest of the day, such as the majority of the population do! They would have wandered all day, built, climbed, killed and maybe run for a couple of minutes here and there. It was a continuous flow of movement. A far cry from the way we live our lives today. We need to 'move it, move it!'

When you exercise it's important to ensure you use five specific movements, squatting, pushing, pulling, lifting and lunging but also to use these five movements in balance. For example, too much pushing and not enough pulling will end up with tightening and shortening of the muscles in the front of your body as well as lengthening and weakening the muscles in the back. Like everything in life – there is an importance for balance in exercise!

However, here is a little gem to make you smile and love me more than ever. Too much exercise can be bad for your health. Ha ha ha! I saw that huge grin wash over your entire face and I am sure I have your attention now. This woman is on your side my friend, are you beginning to realise this yet? Yes, next time your skinny buddy with the washboard stomach gloats about the endless hours pushing herself to the point of exhaustion in the gym, you can smile(inwardly because it is more polite,) knowing that the physical demands she is choosing to place on her body is not exactly ensuring a longer, healthier lifespan than yours. Too much exercise can place extreme stress on the body and in so doing can lower the immune system, close down the reproductive organs and line the heart up for an attack. Moderation is key.

In my view one of the worst exercise related statements is 'no pain, no gain.' I mean, come on, who wants to inflict mental and physical pain and suffering onto themselves especially when both mind and body already work so hard in this life? (I must admit, when I was a young ballet dancer there was nothing I liked more than to feel pain after the intense training. If I didn't have pain, I believed I had not worked hard enough. More recently I was told by my chiropractor, the worst possible people for not recognising pain were dancers, because they learn how to ignore it and move through it. It is not the best way to be. Whoops!) We need the sensation of pain to let us know when our bodies need extra care and it's an important signal, one we should listen to and not ignore. When you hurt yourself exercising it is usually the muscle that hurts as it gets damaged, which then needs rest so that it can heal. Maybe one day, or two or even more, which in my mind is self- defeating when it comes to exercise continuity! And from a psychological point of view, if something hurts you, you tend not to do it again because you remember the pain and how uncomfortable you felt. It is much better to exercise in moderation, without the pain and with all the gain.

Like other stressors in our lives such as a lack of sleep, emotional stress, poor nutritional intake, poor lifestyle choices — exercise can directly affect the body's complex immune system and produce inflammatory responses. Health is ultimately about controlling inflammation which is generally part of a healthy immune response; however, sometimes this process becomes uncontrolled if the insult on inflammation continues over a period of time. This may lead to a state of chronic inflammation that can trigger the development of diseases such as cancer. Thus it makes sense to control the amount of inflammation we inflict upon our bodies, as and where we can. Yes we need to push a little and get exercising because it is health enhancing, but never to the point of causing continuous inflammation or it defeats the object completely by making us sick!

Some foods, such as chips, pasta, cheese, cakes, pies and bread, and most things processed, provoke an excessive inflammatory response within your body. Reduce your consumption of these foods to help keep inflammation low. Other foods, such as oily fish, raw spinach, olive oil, broccoli, sweet potato, pineapple, garlic, ginger, turmeric and raw carrots, fight bodily inflammation, so load them up on your plate.

I will admit to you my friend that I was an exercise junkie when I was a dancer. I danced on average 8 hours a day, was a member of a gym where I trained a few days a week and I had swimming lessons to improve my skills and, so I thought, my fitness! I was very mistaken. Over a period of time I became so sick I was forced to quit my thirty two year dance career over -night and spent five years not being able to step inside a gym, let alone dance. It was completely devastating as I danced to live and lived to dance. My body suffered adrenal fatigue (which is a fatigue that is completely debilitating). This had a dominoes effect on my body and led to a thyroid condition known as Hashimoto's disease -an autoimmune disease that attacks the thyroid itself. I lost teeth – which the dentist could not understand as they were not diseased; I had to have three operations on my breasts to deal with horrendous fibrocystic disease and as the specialists called it, 'changing cells' (I was lucky it was not cancer and I am forever grateful); my body was eating its very own muscles for fuel and live muscle tissue was found in my liver to prove it; my muscles became so weak causing me to shake, collapse and be unconscious on occasions. I could no longer climb the stairs at home without having to stop half way to let my legs have a chance to recover, and I was fighting for breath. I could not think properly, rationalise properly, and my memory was very badly affected. It all ended with a mental and physical breakdown and I was generally a complete wreck! Sounds horrendous doesn't it? It was and all because I over exercised, and ate a diet suitable for an anorexic ant, with the stressors of quite a rocky personal life thrown in for good measures! I may also add here, this is where the medical profession seriously let me down and it was two years from my first doctor visit, until my diagnosis, and that only happened because a natural health practitioner told me I had a serious adrenal issue and sent me back to my doctor. OK,I know my own example is not relevant to most people, because dancing was my career, so it meant I exercised many hours each day and most people will exercise for only an hour or so a day....but there are those who do push their body beyond reasonable limits.....could you be one? If so be warned about the unnecessary stress you put on your body by over exercising. I am proof that over exercise is bad for you and am now proof that moderate exercise is fabulous for you!

So there is a little warning about over exercising, but

my friend, (this is where I hope the glow of love for me will not go out in a flash) too little exercise, or none at all, is bad for you too! Stay with me.....

Couch potatoes are more likely to suffer aching joints, lower moods, fatty organs, obesity, high cholesterol, heart attacks, diabetes type 2, and generally poor health which can result in serious disease. So let there be no confusion here as to whether or not you need to exercise, because you do! Do you still love me? No matter, don't give up and keep reading.

You see, if we go back to our ancestors again, they would have been on the move all day, walking, wandering or having a couple of short sprinting bursts. They would have squatted, lunged, pushed, pulled and lifted each day too. This is, therefore, in our genetic make -up. We are not designed to sit for hours on end in front of the TV, computer, or behind the wheel of a car. We are meant to keep moving...all day. If you do not continue to move as part of your lifestyle, then as you get older you will become stiffer in your movement and even simple tasks such as getting out of bed in the morning, will become more difficult and painful. The older you get, the less you will be able to physically do. And as for climbing the stairs, your lungs and your heart will be so out of shape that the physical exertion of climbing will be almost too much to deal with!

So if too much exercise is bad, and too little exercise is bad, what is the answer? Moderate exercise at lower intensities is the better course. However as with diet, and clothes, there is not a one size fits all plan for exercise and you must find the one that suits you. You need to build up your strength slowly, change your exercise routine regularly, rest adequately in between workouts, walk as often as you can, wander as much as you can get away with each day, and not obsess about your programme! Following a moderate exercise programme will give you results which will have you stronger, more flexible and less prone to illness and disease. This is my mantra now and I am very fit and healthy. For me, being strong, fit and curvy beats being super skinny and sick any day!

I want to demonstrate to you how important keeping your body in shape is for your over-all wellbeing, but this I could also write another book about! So, in my uncomplicated fashion, I will highlight one area of the body and hope you get the picture. What part will I choose? The heart? Not this time, I will choose a less obvious one, to really get you thinking. I am sure that you rarely sit on your posterior and think how it plays a major role in your health, so your rear seems like the perfect part for a little focus! Of course we all know that having a well- rounded and beautifully toned butt like Miss Jennifer Lopez, will boost your sex appeal, but working it goes so much further than being able to strut your stuff in your skinny jeans. The three large muscles of your behind - gluteus maximus, gluteus medius and gluteus minimus do more than add a little pertness! These muscles play an important functional role in your body's alignment of the pelvis, torso and legs. Your three glutes are required for virtually every movement carried out by your lower body so keeping them in tip top order will also keep pain at bay in your knees, hips and back (the three most complained about areas for pain). Strong glutes are the engine of your lower body and are important for keeping you on the move. The glute muscles stabilise your pelvis during walking and running, plus strong glutes help with hip extension and forward propulsion. In other words keeping good strong glutes will have you moving about more freely.

And here is another little gem for keeping your rear in good shape and one you would probably never think of –it burns calories for fuel. Isn't that fantastic? Your glutes burn fat and, as such, play a significant role in your weight control! Just think, your glutes have the power to burn that little bit of chocolate you ate last night (not the whole bar though) ….providing, of course, you give them the opportunity! While all muscles act in this way, the gluteal have the greatest potential for burning calories (even at rest) due to their size and mass (you knew big butts were good!). The more muscle you have, the more fat your body is able to burn when you are in a resting state! Amazing, as you are sitting reading this your well- toned butt (I presume you have one?) is burning off the fat for you!

However, if you are suffering from a severe attack of pancake butt, you know, when it's looking a bit flat and just hanging there, or gluteal amnesia (a condition where the glutes become inactive and forget how to work), due to sitting or lying on those lovely large muscles way too much, it is time to get off your derrière and plump it up with a little exercise. Of course not only will you sculpt a better look in your clothes but you will benefit your overall wellbeing with better physiological health, less pain and some very helpful fat burning! Move it and get a kick ass rear view that will work to keep you fit and healthy!

Cecille began a new fitness regime which included going to the gym (her choice) five times a week for an hour at a time. After a few weeks she came to see me to tell me that exercise, although she was enjoying it, was making zero difference to her weight. In fact she had gained a little. Now sometimes you can seemingly gain weight as you turn flab into muscle, as muscle weighs more than fat, which is why I always advise my clients to take their vital measurements and not solely rely on the scales. However, our conversation uncovered the fact that Cecille was making a common mistake with her exercise regime. She was eating a huge meal after each gym session, because she had 'earnt it'.Cecille was managing to munch her way through a good 800 calories in one meal, and not 800 calories of the best food choices either. I asked her to check the amount of calories she was burning in the gym. She did and she was burning around 380! She did the maths. This is a common error of thinking and you only have to look around the café area of any gym to see the error in full flow! I am sure you would not be one to make this error my friend would you?

I am going to take it that you have got the idea, or are getting the idea as to why exercise is good for you and why you need to incorporate it into your daily life. First up is to find a form of exercise that you will be inspired and motivated to do and that, most importantly, you will enjoy. There is a golden secret form of exercise that ensures exercise need not be tiresome and can be fun. Yes, fun. You know where you enjoy it, laugh during it, and feel fabulous after it (bring anything to mind?). Are you burning to know what this brilliant, golden secret form of exercise is? OK, because it is you, I will share the golden secret…. see still on your side, still sharing the love my friend………The golden secret exercise is….drum roll……. whatever it is that makes you move around that you enjoy. That is so very simple isn't it? Of course enjoyment will vary from person to person, but that is the golden secret and it will produce motivated and inspired exercise, which is exactly what you want and need.

I will be predictable now - doesn't happen too often so you are honoured, and I will list some exercise examples that may inspire or motivate you to break out into a flurry of movement. I will start off with the obvious and then move onto the things perhaps you would not have considered to be exercise. Just remember exercise merely means to move it, raise your heartbeat, challenge your muscles a little and have a bit of fun!

The human body was born to walk (as you have already read) but although a leisurely stroll is better than sitting on your couch, a push to walk at a faster pace to achieve a moderate intensity level will be more beneficial to your overall health . Remember you need to get your heart beating a little faster so walk with a determined stride. Walking up and down a few slight inclines will challenge you even more, so do your best to choose a walk with a few in it. Remember, our ancestor's would have walked all day, so you should incorporate as much walking as you can into your day. A great way to see how much you walk, or how much you don't walk, is to invest in a pedometer. Wear it for a week and be surprised at what you do. You should be achieving 10,000 steps a day on average...... I wonder what you are achieving?

I am happy to be indulging in my now, almost daily, home sessions of yoga, a form of exercise I turned my nose up at when I was dancing - although the floor bar exercises we use to do had some similarities! Ignorance is not always bliss! Yoga helps strengthen your muscles, keeps you flexible, aids circulation and creates a calm feeling in your body and mind. In fact here are a few more benefits: If you regularly practice yoga this will help lower your pulse rate and boost cardiac health. Yoga also decreases the respiratory rate through a combination of controlled breathing exercises, massages internal organs, and helps the body to have a balanced metabolism .Yoga stimulates the detoxification process within the body and provides energy and improves posture and core strength. It reduces anxiety as well as providing an over- all feeling of well -being. Enough reasons for you to give it a go? Nothing to lose, (except, perhaps, a little trapped wind !) and everything to gain.

Swimming a few lengths or participating in Aqua classes will not only raise your heart rate and improve your heart health, the water provides multi-directional resistance that will improve your muscular strength and tone. The increased buoyancy supplies support to the body and decreases the strain placed on weight-bearing joints which makes water based exercise easier and more comfortable for those who may be pregnant, those of us who are a little older, those carrying excess kilos and those physically less able or injured. You could have some swimming lessons to improve your stroke and your breathing because when you do, swimming will become much easier and it is always good to know how to swim properly so you can impress the other half (and on lookers around the pool) on holiday!

However, if you are seeking something a little more challenging than walking and swimming try hiking, cycling, or, dancing. Join a club to play hockey, netball, ping pong, five a side football; or learn to rock climb, horse ride, sail or play tennis (could you be the next Wimbledon Champion?). Stretch out that body with some health balancing yoga, and tone muscles at a Pilates class. There are so many forms of exercise on offer these days, and if you spend some time looking into it you will probably find something that you will enjoy.

Now let's look at forms of exercise you may not have thought about or have considered as exercise. There are many cheap activities that you can do on your own that don't involve equipment or technical expertise and you can bring the family together and enjoy time with the kids. How about rounders' in the park with all the family avec un grand picnic, or playing chase or hide and seek with the kids? How about a little sticky toffee (do you remember that?) or a game of Bulldog? Get some friends to join you with their families and play relay races and team games on the beach or in the park. Walk the kids to school with the new dog – dogs are a marvellous excuse to walk, come rain or shine, they're a companion for you whilst you do walk and obviously your best friend too. Take the kids swimming and play games in the pool like they do – let them lead the way. Children have oodles of play energy which we forget how to use as we get older. They know how to have fun and laugh which is fabulous exercise for the entire body. The best thing of all is that kids seemingly never tire (so true yes?) – thus the challenge is to keep up with them! Include even more fun and laughter and have a game of twister, this will have you stabilising your core muscles as you try not to fall over and clenching those gluteus maximus muscles on and off to refrain from letting dangerous gases escape.

If you don't have kids to play with, and you don't fancy borrowing one or two, what can you do alone that does not involve the gym fees? I am a great fan of exercising outside, so why not get a few friends together and play football, or rounders, or cricket in the local park. This is great fun and something we have always done as a family. (Rather embarrassing, a couple of years ago we were having a big family game of cricket and my dad ran me out. He was eighty six years old!)There are plenty of outdoor exercise programmes to join if you want to be part of a class or group. If the weather is not so great, you could crank up the music good 'n loud and get boogying to your favourite tracks whilst doing the housework at high intensity, or dance like crazy naked or otherwise, as you are getting ready for work in the morning (Just be sure to close the curtains if you do the naked bit!).Music is very motivational and inspirational and will be sure to get you moving. And talking of music, it is wonderfully social and quite the fashion at the moment to brush up that soft shoe shuffle and 'Come Dancing'. You never know, you may find your Cinderella or Prince Charming whilst learning to Cha Cha or your Fred Astaire or Ginger Rogers, when tapping those feet. Or try a completely different form of dancing – Like Pole dancing, or belly dancing, which will bring you a core strength to be envious of, and sexy moves that will raise….. your self -esteem.

If you like to work out in the privacy of your home, there are many DVDs out there offering 10 minute workout programmes which are easy to fit into your day, and although I would say don't be misled by the picture of the body on the front of the box, you can tone up well using a variation of these throughout your week. You could invest a few pounds in a rebounder – a small version of a trampoline, and bounce your way to good health whilst watching your favourite TV show – which is a win win situation is it not?

Offering a dog walking service is a great way to get fit and earn a few extra pennies without the responsibility of having a mutt full time. It is a way to get paid to get fit! But if you are seeking something with a little more adrenaline rush than the neighbour's Rover can offer you, how about giving paddle boarding a go?. It's not quite kayaking and it's not quite surfing… stand up paddle boarding is a sea sport where you stand on a long board and manoeuvre with a large paddle. It's a real muscle work out and it's great for improving your core strength and balance – I am not speaking from personal participation here, just what others have said! Plus you get to enjoy being out in the fresh air and soaking up the sun, (for an extra vitamin D hit) that's if it's not raining!

If you are in to gardening, or even if you are not, time how long it takes you to get the job done. Note this down as your personal best. Then mow the lawn and dig the garden quicker than usual and each time you do, try to break your personal best. Offer to keep the neighbours garden, or an elderly relatives too and enjoy the extra workout and feel good factor of helping someone else. You never know, this may also end in getting paid to be fit too!

Do you remember playing with a hula hoops in the gym or playground at Primary school? I bet that brings back memories! There you were in your cute little PE kit, swinging your hips with all your might, trying to keep the hula hoop around your waist. Could it be time to invest in your very own hula hoop and get twisting your way to fitness once again (with or without the cute PE kit)? There are many classes out there as well as teach yourself DVDs to help get you hula hooping once again. I am sure you will spend a fair amount of time giggling like crazy which, as you know, is also fabulous exercise for your body and mind.

Most people lack enough discipline to stick to an exercise programme alone, and choosing to get fit with a friend, or two, has huge motivational benefits, plus it can be a lot more fun. Find yourself an exercise buddy if you feel you would benefit from having someone else to train with. Laugh as you work out and it will double the great effects of exercise. I use to train with a client in a gym and we would sometimes have to stop and compose ourselves we would laugh so much! Always have some fun whilst exercising and you will cease to see it as a chore.

And talking of exercise buddies here's one last

suggestion for some great adult exercise - have lots of sex, wild or otherwise!!!It is a complete body and mind workout, and will leave you with a fabulously, healthy after- glow. It boosts the immune system, lowers your blood pressure, improves pelvic floor muscles to reduce incontinence (which around 30% of women will suffer from at some point in their lives) and keeps your oestrogen and testosterone levels in balance. Sex also eases stress (maybe I should have included this in my Stress management program?!), and orgasms can block pain such as headaches (no excuses ladies!), back, leg and in some cases, arthritic pain! And as we all know, great sex induces some jolly good sleep - just do your best not to snore immediately after as it kind of kills the romance of the moment!

Go on admit it, there was at least one form of exercise there that inspired you, even if it was just a quick flicker!

There is every reason to engage in moderate exercise, and there are only poor excuses not to. Exercise will keep you younger, flexible, happier, healthier and less prone to serious disease. It will enhance your energy to live and enjoy a wonderful life. On the opposite side of the coin, not exercising will leave you prone to being stiff, with excess fat, a sluggish metabolism and at a much higher risk of serious disease. Not really a question of what is best or what makes better sense is it?

OK, I may have convinced you that it is good for your overall wellbeing to exercise, that you do not need to join a gym, unless you want to and that you can have fun exercising, but just how much do you need to do? The other big excuse not to exercise is time. Everyone is too busy. They would exercise for sure if they had time…but they just do not have any spare time. Amazing how some of us manage to squeeze it into our day, perhaps we live a less busy or demanding life!!! Ha ha! It is probably that we realise the importance of exercise, feel the difference when we do and prioritise it into our day.

People often ask me what my personal work out programme consists of these days. Well for starters, don't expect something mega! I mix it up good and proper over the week, with no two days the same. The only consistency is the walking. I walk my dog two – three times a day for between twenty and forty minutes each time (any longer and my hips become uncomfortable). I play games with my dog every day too…footie, or tug or just fetch. I do between ten and twenty minutes of weights, kettle bell, swiss ball, twist plate, rebounder, or dance (or a combination thereof), followed by some yoga stretches and some floor bar that I use to do when I danced. Some days I may do just my yoga, and I always have a day off each week…except from the dog walking – not sure she would appreciate a day off! In the summer I swim nearly every day and workout in the pool or sea. If I am in the UK I may go to the gym with my son, or get thrashed in a game of tennis with him! A real mixed bag…. but I am always moving. You will rarely see me sitting still. And as for sex………..

If you have children, you can schedule in play time with them, where you play active games together. Get them off the computer, and away from the PlayStation, and have some fun and games before dinner. Not only will you all be healthier, but playing together will strengthen bonds between you. Using being a parent as an excuse not to exercise has no merit. Like I said, playing games is fabulous exercise and can be done during the week and at weekends. Better to not clean the house, or leave the dishes, or ditch the ironing, than to pass up on the chance of playing with your babes. Bike rides, and games in the park will have you all smiling with the benefits and your exercise is done!

What to eat before and after you exercise? This is advice for the novice exerciser, not the athlete.....A light workout is perfectly fine on an empty stomach, but if you feel you need to eat before you do, keep it light and do not train after a heavy meal! Try a good quality protein shake, or a banana and a handful of nuts, or a couple of oat cakes with nut butter or some mashed avocado. After, make sure you reverse the effects of free radicals which would have been released during exercise and you repair muscles by eating lots of foods which contain vitamin C, E, selenium and copper, such as fruits, nuts, seeds, vegetables whole grains and a little protein.

Ok, so you don't have kids, or you have teenagers who would rather do a bungee jump over a crocodile infested river, than be seen exercising with mum or dad. Get up 10 minutes earlier, and do a simple workout regime 5 days a week. 10 minutes – that is not too much to ask, so don't start firing excuses as to why you need those extra 10 minutes in bed. If you are fit and healthy, you will be bouncing out from under the covers refreshed and raring to go in the mornings, and if you are not, time to get your body moving to bring you to this heavenly state. There are many 10 minute (and less) work out DVD or YouTube options to help you on your way, but if that is not your thing, go for a 10 minute bike ride or brisk walk, skip for ten minutes, walk up and down your stairs for 10 minutes, do 10 minutes of star jumps and alternate leg lunges, 10 minutes on a rebounder, or the trampoline, 10 minutes between a twist plate and balance board or start your day with a 10 minute stretch. Do four minutes of cardio, (jumping up and down on the rebounder, or star jumps – anything to raise your heartbeat) and 1 minute of lifting weights - times two - and you have your 10 minutes busted! There are numerous options for you to try, it is a matter of finding what you enjoy most. Mix it up over the week to keep it fresh and be inventive with your programme. A short blast of energy can have a lasting effect on metabolism for the entire day and a regular exercise practice, even if it's just 10 minutes, can have a lasting impact on heart health and mental acuity. Got to be worth those 10 minutes and it would be even better if you could fit in a second session a day!

If you join a tennis club or a martial arts group, or a line dancing programme or you have the rose clasped firmly between your teeth for your Tango class (or something similar) you will probably be exercising for an hour once a week. You need to aim for 3 times a week at this level, so find a practice buddy or combine it with one of the other suggestions above. Joining clubs and classes has social benefits and the chances are you will make new friends. These will be friends who share your interest and this in itself is motivational.

We all live too much of a sedentary life these days. What with computers, cars, TV, internet shopping, we have little reason to get up off our backsides, which we know we need to keep in good shape! Nevertheless, no matter how sedentary your life is, it will pay you dividends to move every hour at least once – remember our ancestors would be on the move all day. Jump up from your office chair and walk around, looking important, of course. Get moving during the commercial breaks on the TV (after all it is far more beneficial to avoid all the processed food they are trying to sell you), embarrass the kids and have a quick boogie to the tune on the radio, get out of your car at the next service station and walk around the entire perimeter. Whenever possible, move every hour or, even better, every 10 minutes if you can. Sitting halts the muscle activity that is important to aid processes that break down fats and sugars within the body. If you are not breaking down fats and sugars you put your-self at a higher risk of things such as heart disease and diabetes type 2. It is even said that standing instead of sitting is better for your health and burns a few more calories an hour. So why not try standing for a while as part of your daily exercise programme too? That is easy exercise. Simply stand and work at the computer....I am standing as I write this. So move around every hour for a minute or a two, and stand whenever possible rather than sitting. Simple, easy and your body will thank you.

Ask yourself a couple of questions - How else can you get moving during your day that you can build into your lifestyle? Or how could you build on something that's already part of your routine? Walking to work, or walking during your lunch break are easy options and that boost of fresh air and, hopefully, sunshine, will lift your mood and boost your vitamin D levels too. You may even find the afternoon slump in the office disappears and you have better focus for the rest of the day. Could you ride your bike to work or to do the local errands? Take the stairs instead of the lift. Go from sitting to standing to sitting again, 10 times in a row. (Rest for a minute, then repeat.)Walk around whilst talking on your mobile phone. Get off the bus a stop early or park at the far end of the car park so you have to walk a little more. Anyhow you can, fit in some extra moving around.

When I fly between countries I will be the one at the airport who takes the stairs, not the escalator, who walks to the departure lounge at a pace, and not on the moving walkways, who stands whilst waiting to be called onto the plane and who moves her legs, neck, shoulders and arms every so often whilst on the plane (being careful not to poke my neighbours as I do or kick the seat of the person in front!) I will even visit the loo an extra time just to walk and stand in a queue! There is enough time for sitting on the aeroplane, the rest of the time is for moving.

Getting fitter and leaner requires a bit of a plan, otherwise it would be too easy to get side tracked and go off course. You need to be clear about your aims and what you wish to achieve from them. Setting yourself a goal is a great idea, but make it achievable, -challenging but achievable, or you will lose enthusiasm and be more likely to give up. You need to give your goal a time frame otherwise it has no end! And then chunk it into bite size pieces, smaller goals if you like, and as you achieve these smaller steps have a reward system in place.

This is likely to keep you motivated as you tick each small goal off on your way to the jackpot and rewarding yourself as you do will help you realise how well you are doing.

S tinky was three stone overweight, had blood pressure issues, was 'border line' (I don't do borderline... you either have or you do not...but hey....the medical profession does border lines!) diabetic and had high cholesterol. We started nice and slow. In the UK I have a toning table, which is a table you lie on and it does exercises for you by moving your body. That may sound a bit lazy, and it was primarily introduced for easy inch loss, but it offers great physiotherapy and gets a very stiff body moving without the person having to do much other than lie there. (It is very good for those who are very unfit, with Multiple Sclerosis, ME, and physical disabilities). So Stinky started with sessions on the toning table and gradually we introduced some walking, a couple of minutes on a rebounder, a little exercise bike, some twist plate and a couple of minutes using a step. Over a period of six months Stinky lost a stone and a half, reduced his blood pressure and cholesterol and was told he was no longer considered borderline diabetic (he did not have diabetes). We worked at his diet (although he had a very social working life and ate in restaurants most days) and he did take some supplements, but the exercise paid off. Stinky felt a lot more lithe, less stressed, and younger! And of course, his health was in much better shape.

Of course you could make your exercise beneficial for charity, by getting fit in time for a charitable event or asking people to sponsor you and what you make donate to charity. These are great forms of motivation and you will have others watching your progress which will inspire you to keep going.

Agree your goal with a friend, this will work to hold you to it and turns it into a challenge. Pin your written goal up where you can see it as this will keep you focused. Visualise your success. Have a clear mental picture in your mind of how you will look and feel once you have achieved your goal. Take a couple of minutes each day to visualise and go through various scenarios, such as walking up stairs, or playing football in the garden with the kids and feel how fit and capable you are. Visualise yourself in that little black dress looking stunning and in shape, or see yourself jog along the beach in your speedos. Visualise yourself going to the doctor and having better health test results. See the amazement on the doctor's face and feel the smug smirk on yours!!

Take photographs of yourself at the beginning and then at intervals, such as every four weeks, so you can track your progress. Measure your vital statistics and write them up each week to see how your body tones up and where you may need to pay extra attention. Have a training partner, but if you can't find one, consider hiring a personal trainer, (which need be only at four week intervals again if you can't afford one every week), as this will also help to keep you on track.

And if after all this you would rather remain snuggled up under the duvet in the mornings than get exercising before your day begins, OK. But whilst you lay there have a little stretch. Stretch long and tall and then release, and then stretch in a star shape and repeat each movement a few times. Stretching will increase circulation and oxygen to the muscles, improve flexibility and should help you to wake up less grumpily than normal!

Whatever exercise you do, it should complement the type of person you are. If you suffering from fatigue, don't start with hard and fast training my friend….it is the worst thing you could do. If you are pregnant, don't start a complicated work-out routine if you were not doing this before you were pregnant. If you are already quite physically fit, look into how you can take it up a notch or two. If you are very over weight, or sick perhaps seek professional advice before you embark on a new exercise plan and check with your GP. Like any change, slowly, slowly does it. If you are a beginner, start with the walking and aim to walk for between ten and fifteen minutes each day for two weeks and then increase this to twenty minutes three – five days a week. Within a month this will seem very easy and then you can decide what else you are going to include in your plan to increase the benefits. Remember if you cause pain you will not gain….so be clever about what you do. Even though I may have inspired you to exercise and you are extremely excited, please don't go running five kilometres straight off….you may end up hospitalised, which is not the aim! Slow, steady, progress will get you there…I promise.

If you are still really put off by the word exercise, replace the word. Replace it with the word fun, and ask yourself 'What form will your fun take today?' Then go have some fun!

Shall I end this with telling you the absolutely undisputed, best exercise you can ever do? Yes I think I should be fair, you have read all this so you deserve to know. Sorry to have kept this from you until the end, but as my mother has always said, it is good to save the best to last. The best exercise is…..the one you will do!!!

Walk, run, climb, play, you can do it! Exercise means moving it so your heart beat rises and you challenge your muscles, but within moderation. Exercise can be and should be fun, you just need to find the form you enjoy and maybe find an exercise buddy to enjoy it with, or get all the family involved. Exercise at least 3 times a week, and it needn't be for hours on end. Move around every hour or more when you can. Stand instead of sitting and walk as much as you can, even if it is around the house! Remember to include the five basic movements: squatting, pushing, pulling, lifting and lunging where you can. There, that isn't so bad now is it? It can all slot nicely into your lifestyle if you choose to let it. So what fun will you chose to start with? Whatever you do, start to move and feel the benefits that go with it. All that and no mention of Lycra, treadmills, sweat or exhaustion – just fun and plenty of it!

Supplements

"Ask not what you can do for your country. Ask what's for lunch." — Orson Welles

In my role as a nutritionist, my first concern is with the quality of the food we eat and sustaining a healthy disposition by eating an optimum diet. However there are times when diet or health is compromised and it is necessary to boost nutrients by supplementation. There is an argument I hear all too often, that if we eat a good diet, there should be no reason to take supplements. Of course, I would be the first to agree with this whole heartedly, after all, who really wants to be popping pills all day? And supplementation would not be necessary if only we followed a healthy, well balanced diet, lived in a toxin free environment and were never sick or under the influence of stress.

So why use supplements? There are a host of reasons why it is good to take a course of supplements alongside our diet, but I will keep it uncomplicated as per the title of this book and give you a brief outline:

Let's start by looking at the foodstuffs themselves: commercial agricultural techniques have meant our fruit and vegetables are often grown in nutrient deficient soils, and as a consequence our food is often also nutrient deficient. Many foods are shipped long distances (especially fruit and vegetables) and can be stored for long periods of time. Both of these factors lead to the depletion of vital nutrients, including the important B-complex and C vitamins. Then when food is processed, cooked, or preserved there is further nutrient depletion. By the time it gets to your plate it is already seriously compromised when it comes down to what good it will do you and it will do little to help you in your quest for great health. There is also the fact that many unnatural things are added to our food such as preservatives, sugar, salt, unhealthy fats and hormones which need to be dealt with internally by our bodies and eliminated successfully, which cannot, and does not, always happen if we are nutrient deficient.

From the human being's perspective; we do tend to nurture some erratic eating habits- for example, generally we don't chew our food sufficiently (most of the time because we are eating on the run);, as I have mentioned earlier we do not always eat a balanced diet, and we can be under stress which contributes to poor digestion (see my chapter on Stress). All this makes it difficult for our bodies to extract the full spectrum of nutrients it needs from food. A vast amount of people take medication which can deplete essential nutrients, and at certain times in our lives, such as when we are pregnant for instance, or if we are ill, we need to increase certain nutrients to aid health. Some of us may have genetic weaknesses, which require us to have more of a certain nutrient.

Environmentally, we suffer from pollution in our air, water and food and as a consequence our body needs more nutrients than normal to eliminate the toxins safely from our system. Quite often our body needs a helping hand to detox which can be aided by supplementation.

So having outlined briefly foodstuffs, human and environmental factors, can you see why there may be a need to supplement your diet in order to enjoy great health? However, my friend, as one who believes in balance, I am not of the belief that we all need to supplement all the time. Like I have said, who would want to be popping pills all the time, be it drugs or natural supplements? Indeed if we could only learn to listen to when our bodies are screaming at us for help, as they do, or we could anticipate the need for extra nutrients, such as the onset of winter, or a particular stressful time in our lives such as a wedding, then we could learn when to supplement successfully (in advance even better as this is the true practice of prevention rather than cure) without feeling the need to do so every day for the rest of our lives.

As it was with our diet, the question is where to begin with supplementation. There is an array of supplements out there and it can be quite challenging to know which one to pick. They line the shelves of the health shops, the pharmacies and the supermarkets and there are also plenty to choose from on the internet. The question is though, what are the right ones for you? How can you choose between brands and different supplements? I mean, do you need a B-Complex, or a course of Milk Thistle? Do you need a multi-vitamin for 50 plus, even though you are 49 years old, or just a Vitamin C top up? It can be very complicated when you are standing in front of the shelves!

And again, as it is with your diet, any supplements you choose to take should be healthy too. What is required is cost effective, high potency nutritional support that is in a chelated form (pronounced, keylated), which means the body can utilise it. It is always a great shame to waste your hard earned cash on something you may as well cut out the middle man with (you!) and throw directly down the toilet because your body cannot use it effectively. You need a supplement that is gentle on the stomach, is complete and comprehensive and does not contain allergens such as yeast, dairy, gluten, lactose, soya, sugar, artificial sweeteners, preservatives and colours, which your body may not react kindly to. You need a supplement that will provide the nutrient is says it does on the box, in a powerful form that will boost your body's natural stores. Wow, you may say, that is one heck of a supplement, but aren't they all like that? Errrrrghhhh......no!!!! All supplements are not created equal my friend. I cringe when I see some of the additives, and shake my head in despair when I see some of the levels of nutrients! There are some very poor supplements out there on the shelves, but you are not to know that unless you are an expert, like moi! You will not find many consumer products, apart from cigarettes, marketed as 'Not that good for you' and it would be counter- productive for the manufacturer in the main, if supplements were marketed in this way!

Good supplement companies will give you details about the quality and an extensive amount of information on the label. Check to see if the ingredients are pesticide free, whether or not they are tested on animals, are suitable if you are a vegan and if they are free from artificial sweeteners, preservatives and colours. (The last thing you want is a hyper active child because they have ingested a vitamin that is full of E numbers and sugar!)If you are buying fish oils, for instance my friend, it is essential to ensure the company makes statements about the purity and stability of the product and guarantees they are free from mercury and PCBs. You would not want to be swallowing an unwanted dose of mercury! The best companies will take pride in providing the highest quality nutritional supplements money can buy and many will back that up with a money back scheme if you are not satisfied with their products. These are the kind of companies I work with, and the health results I see in my clients are amazing.

Prairie Dawn came to see me about her depression, her under active thyroid (which, even though she was on Thyroxin for, she still felt she suffered the many symptoms of), her pre-menstrual mood swings and her weight issues. Apart from a change in diet I suggested that she embarked on a course of supplements which included the full spectrum of my protocol: a multivitamin - but one designed to support thyroid function - an Omega 3 fish oil, a digestive enzyme and a probiotic. At first Prairie Dawn was not on board with the suggestion as she had previously taken a course of supplements recommended by her doctor. As is often the case, the doctor (who remember does not have intense training in nutrition) had not recommended any more than a vitamin C supplement and an Evening Primrose oil both of which were of a low dose and not what I would call a 'clean' supplement – without additives. Prairie Dawn had taken these for a month without noticing a single difference to her health and so had brushed them aside - along with her belief in any supplements being of any use at all. In the end, with gentle persuasion and the promise of a refund from the supplement company if the supplements did not work, Prairie Dawn began her program. After just three days she contacted me to say she felt oddly different, like a weight had been taken off her shoulders and asked me if this could be the supplements. I told her it was hard to tell, as it was a little soon for me to judge results, but was of course happy she felt lighter. After three weeks she contacted me again to tell me she was positively happy, had lost three kilos in weight, was sleeping like a baby and had an energy she had forgotten she could have. She was also able to go to the toilet every day (she had been suffering constipation for a very long while), and her skin on her face was clearing from some unsightly red blotches she had. After three further months on her program Prairie dawn felt in tiptop health and, much to the delight of her family, had not suffered any pre- menstrual mood swings! As a result of how well she was feeling we reduced her protocol down to a general multi vitamin and the fish oil – still alongside a healthy diet, of course. Two years on she is a strong advocate of how a healthy diet and the correct supplement program has helped her regain her physical and mental health. As a result her whole family are on a multi-vitamin and fish oil program throughout the winter months to boost their immune system and their mental state which Prairie Dawn says works wonders!

So what supplements should you take? Of course a lot depends upon the results you are looking for, and the state of your current health, but in my practice I have a general protocol that I follow with my clients if they are looking to improve health. Of course, we are all individual and everyone needs specific nutrient combinations, but for the most part, everyone will benefit immensely from - a comprehensive Multi Vitamin, an Essential Omega Oil, Probiotic and Digestive Enzyme. There are specialist cases where I recommend targeted formulas, of course, but as a rule of thumb it is all about rebalancing the body and helping the digestive system to work to optimum levels, so that the body has the necessary tools to do the job itself. This is my way of working, and I have seen incredible outcomes by using this simple programme....after all life is only as complicated as you choose to make it! And as this book is supposed to be an uncomplicated guide, I will not stun you with talk about all the various supplements you COULD take. Let's keep this simple as promised my friend.

I will now offer you a little on each of my protocol supplements so you understand my program and how you may benefit from it.

Multi vitamins

Vitamins and minerals are essential for life – they boost the immune system, support normal growth and development, and help cells and organs do their work. The correct vitamins can combat your sugar cravings, lower your cholesterol levels, reduce your risk of heart disease and even enhance your sex life! Woohoo! If you become deficient your health will suffer in one way or another. For example, if you are deficient in vitamin C you can suffer from bleeding gums, blood clots in veins, coughs, colds, viruses etc. If you are deficient in iodine you can suffer from hypothyroidism, lack of energy and poor fat metabolism. As I have discussed earlier, most of us will have a nutritional deficiency somewhere along the line because of our diet, lifestyle and even genetics.

Vitamin C must be one of the most well -known nutrients. It is a nutrient that we cannot make for ourselves. We need an average (and that is average, which, of course, none of us are!) of 300mg a day – that's about 6 oranges, unless you are sick, have bleeding gums, wrinkles, poor immunity or smoke, in which case you need much higher amounts. So you can munch your way through a sack of oranges a day (best done whilst sitting on the toilet, as it saves the run)....or take a supplement.

Each vitamin and mineral will be reliant on another in order to be absorbed or used effectively. For example you need vitamin D to absorb calcium, you need all the B vitamins in balance, so that the body can use them effectively. That is why it is necessary for any supplement you take to be correctly balanced and comprehensive. If you are short on one nutrient, it can have a knock on effect throughout your entire body. This is why I prefer to recommend a full spectrum multi vitamin rather than individual vitamins, unless I am consulting on a specific case which may require a different approach. And this is a safer option for you too, as guessing which one vitamin may help you, may lead to other deficiencies or you may even choose the wrong vitamin altogether.

A daily multi-vitamin, is a good way to ensure you're

aiming in the right direction to obtain all the nutrients you need to live a fit and healthy existence. It can help fill in the gaps, so to speak, and it is an excellent, inexpensive insurance policy for your health. Like any dietary supplements, multivitamins are meant to be taken alongside a healthy diet to supplement the nutrients required by the body. Eating a well- balanced diet and taking a quality supplement will ensure a more beneficial outcome with greater results, but that is not to say that you cannot take them, indeed you should, if your diet is in need of an overhaul!

> Lacking in energy? There could be all kinds of reasons why, but perhaps you are running low in, and need a boost of B vitamins and Magnesium......or vitamin C, or D....or........

We need a complete range of vitamins and minerals daily to function and evidence has shown that having a diet that is over the RDA (recommended daily amount – which by the way is the bare minimum required to survive, and not necessarily the amount you need to be fit, well and bursting with energy!) may also prevent age-related disease. This means protection for you against diseases such as osteoporosis, dementia, and cardiac problems.

Multi vitamins come in various forms: for males and females, and to help during pregnancy. You will find them in tablet or drink form, pastilles, chewable, and those specially formulated for children. However, if you are not consulting with a professional who knows about vitamins and minerals, and may I add, you are very welcome to contact me for advice, you need to look out for all the points I have mentioned. I am serious when it comes to quality and so should you be – after all, you are worth it!

During the short, dark winter days, it can be difficult to spend enough time outdoors in daylight for your body to produce the right amounts of vitamin D. Vitamin D deficiency can lead to low moods. Supplementing your diet may see improvements in your mood and well-being.

"50,000-63,000 individuals in the United States and 19,000-25,000 in the UK die prematurely from cancer annually due to insufficient vitamin D."
— John Cannell

The Omega oils – Omega 3,6 and 9

It is crucial to include the essential fatty acids, 3 and 6 in your diet because the body itself cannot produce them, which is why they are known as essential. Omega-3s and omega-6s have very important roles in maintaining cells, are needed for the synthesis of prostaglandins, which help regulate blood clotting, body temperature, blood pressure, reproduction and immune function. These wonderful oils have been well studied for their role in the support of many systems in the body including the brain and inflammation.

Did you know that 60% of your brain and the nerves that run all over your body are made up of fats? This means we need to ensure they continue to get a good supply of quality fats. It stands to reason that the better the fat the body ingests, the better your brain and nerves will work. It also stands to reason that if you are not getting enough of the right fats, your brain will suffer. Yes, forget about remembering where your keys are, you may not remember where your house is and you will certainly forget where you parked your car! We need good, healthy fats. The low fat diet fads out there have been responsible for a huge amount of people starving themselves of essential fats because they have been led to believe that all fat is bad and will make them sick and fat. These people have not understood that fat is necessary, in the right form, for good health and in fact can keep you nice and slim!

In today's diet, many people consume way too much Omega 6, found in refined vegetable oils, especially soy oil, which is used in fast foods, and processed foods including biscuits, cakes and sweeties. Hormones derived from omega-6 fatty acids tend to increase inflammation (an important component of the immune response), blood clotting, and cell proliferation, which is particularly unhelpful for us all, health conscious or not! Too much Omega 6 can make you fat and hence put you at risk of chronic diseases, but we do need Omega 6 as I first said. Omega-6 fatty acids play a crucial role in brain function, as well as normal growth and development. Also known as polyunsaturated fatty acids (PUFAs), they help stimulate skin and hair growth, maintain bone health, regulate metabolism, and maintain the reproductive system.

Houston, we have a problem. For as many people as there are who eat too much Omega 6 in their diet , there are just as many people who do not eat enough Omega 3 found mainly in the fat of oily fish such as salmon, sardines, herring, mackerel, and tuna. Also known as polyunsaturated fatty acids (PUFAs), like the omega 6, omega-3 fatty acids play a crucial role in brain function, as well as normal growth and development and they may reduce the risk of heart disease. Fish is something that not everyone likes, or knows how to cook, so is not consumed by the majority of people on a regular basis. (I do my best!) There are plant source omega 3 providers such as walnuts and flaxseeds which contain a precursor omega-3, alpha-linolenic acid (ALA). This can be converted by the body, but can you honestly say that you eat them on a regular basis?

A very worried set of parents bought their 8 year old son, the Two-Headed Monster, to see me. He was behaving very badly at school and was getting into serious trouble. He was also misbehaving a lot at home. The Two-Headed Monster was hyperactive and had very low concentration levels. He bounced around my office and found it very difficult to sit for periods of more than 10 minutes at a time. His diet was pretty good, and lower in sugar than most children who have these kinds of issues. We did alter his diet a little by reducing the amount of meat he was eating. We put him on a specially formulated children's Omega 3 fish oil with vitamin D and E. The change in the Two-Headed Monster was spectacular, even to the point that his teacher wanted to know what magic formula had been used so she could tell other parents about it! The Two-Headed Monster went on to become a model student and a very well behaved child at home.

We need both of the essential fats, Omega 3 and 6, but in the right balance. Once again, here I am harping on about balance!

There is another Omega that is less spoken of, Omega-9, which may benefit health by helping to lower LDL ("bad") cholesterol and raise HDL ("good") cholesterol. Omega 9 may also play a role in controlling blood sugar. So although you do not hear much about number 9, it does play a fairly essential role in your life.

I have witnessed fantastic results after supplementing people who suffer with high cholesterol and blood sugars with Omega oils. I have also seen inflammation lowered, and energy soar, brain function return, and behavioural issues in children corrected, depression lifted, hormones rebalanced, and Multiple Sclerosis symptoms greatly reduced, all by the use of these amazing oils in conjunction with correct diet of course. Way to go, Amigos!

Probiotics

Probiotics are your supply of 'friendly' bacteria. There are 20 times as many bacteria in our bodies as there are cells, which is quite an amazing fact and one that would definitely impress others at your next dinner party! Probiotics balance the gut flora, build the immune system, improve digestion, produce vitamins, such as vitamin K and the B vitamins, lower cholesterol, regulate hormones, and contribute to the health of the colon, hence, as you may well have gathered, they are very important. Without the right amount of 'friendly' bacteria you become wide open to attack by the 'bad' guys. The good bacteria get together and act like a protective shield for your entire body. When I think of probiotics I always remember the scene from the movie 300 when the brave King Leonaidis and his Spartan army were standing side by side, shields poised, waiting fearlessly for battle to begin. I imagine each probiotic as a brave and fearless warrior, fighting by my side to protect me - which is not far from the truth.

Probiotics have long been studied in the treatment of symptoms of IBS (Irritable Bowel Syndrome) and the most commonly studied are Lactobacilli and Bifidobacteria.

However, your friendly bacteria can become compromised and their formidable army reduced in size, when you have been ill, have taken a course of antibiotics, if you use the birth control pill, have had surgery, are under too much stress, are on long term medication, have had infections, suffer from constipation or diarrhoea, have inflammatory bowel conditions, eat a poor diet, or have travelled and suffered from travellers stomach upset. Phew! That sentence needed a big breath! And talking of breath, if you suffer from bad breath, which is not related to a dental issue, you are probably very low on your friendly little fighters too.

I have used probiotics to clear many conditions for my lovely clients, like chest infections, thrush, acne, IBS, Rosacea, upset stomachs, sore throats, cystitis, headaches and indigestion. I have also used them to help strengthen the body of people with more serious diseases such as heart disease, cancer, Crohn's and ME. These potent little supplements give amazing results.

Digestive enzymes

Digestive enzymes break down your food so that your body can assimilate nutrients. Enzymes are a vital part of proper digestion. Incomplete breakdown of food fosters rancid food which causes untold damage as well as digestive complaints. Undigested food impedes the healthy motility function of the colon as it sits there and rots - yuk! If your enzymes were failing to work properly you would have whole chunks of undigested food in your gut, which would be terribly painful and make you sick! Only small particles of food can be absorbed through the gut wall, not large chunks! And as you age your levels of digestive enzymes tend to drop, resulting in more digestive complaints and indigestion after food, as well as general inflammation in the body.

The signs of enzyme deficiency are excess gas, indigestion, heartburn, diarrhoea, and constipation. The body uses a tremendous amount of energy to digest foods that do not contain natural enzymes, such as junk food, and processed foods, and over time this will result in you suffering from depleted energy, declining eyesight, memory loss, allergies and chronic disease. Enzymes are found in fruit and vegetables, but these can be nutrient poor, as we discussed earlier due to growing and cooking techniques. The more raw fruit and vegetables you eat, the better your enzyme levels will become.

I will tell you about a few digestive enzymes and their

functions to help you understand a little more: Amylase breaks down starch, protease breaks down protein, lipase breaks down fat, lactase break down lactose (sugar protein in milk), and cellulose breaks down the fibre of plant cell walls. As you have just read, each enzyme has its own food source that it digests neatly for you. Thus, if you eat a lot of bread, rolls, pies and pasta but have limited supplies of amylase, your digestion of these products will be incomplete, causing you indigestion and other digestive complaints. Ever wondered why you suffered chest pain after eating your lunchtime sandwich?

Enzymes can also be used to support a healthy anti-inflammatory process, which is vital to good health. Enzymes have numerous functions in the body.

Lactase, which breaks down the lactose protein in milk, is one of the best known enzymes, simply because we are aware of lactose intolerance, those who cannot digest milk products. Our stores of lactase are designed to dwindle after we have been weaned, as we are not supposed to drink milk after that age (despite the fact that we think drinking milk is good for us!) leaving us unable to digest the sugar protein in milk. Many people are intolerant and suffer after consuming dairy products, often without realising the cause.

Once digestive enzymes kick into action, digestive systems begin to function effectively again and bodies gain from correct nutrient absorption. Ridding oneself of all the uncomfortable and sometimes, embarrassing, side effects of not having enough enzymes can be a real relief. (A decrease in anti-social wind problems makes for a more relaxed meal out with friends!)Once the enzymes get to work, they instantly spark an improvement in overall health.

As you have read time and time again in this book, your health begins and ends with a healthy gut. Having a gut that works will make a world of difference to anyone. Even if you are taking a quality multivitamin if you have an unhealthy gut this will reduce its beneficial powers, unless the multi-vitamin is one designed for a compromised digestive system (not wishing to add in a complication here). It is for this very reason that my protocol includes digestive aids and if a client is short on funds and cannot afford all four supplements at once, I recommend a course of enzymes and probiotics to rebalance digestion first, and once the digestive system is working satisfactorily, the vitamins and oils – a point worth remembering.

A small word of caution, now that I have got you all psyched up and ready to embark on a course of supplements: There can be contraindications to supplements, especially if you are taking medication, and although you can buy them 'off the shelf', professional advice can never be underestimated and I strongly urge you to seek exactly that when considering a course of supplementation. However, to date, no one has been reported of dying as a result of a vitamin supplement!

And if you do decide to embark on a course of supplements, take them at a different time of the day to any conventional medication.

One last little client story to share with you my friend. Murray is a sports enthusiast. He cycles most days, plays football at the weekends, visits the gym five times a week and often goes 'caving' with his friends (makes me feel claustrophobic and exhausted just thinking about it!). He needed a diet to compliment his high energy lifestyle and wanted to boost it by taking supplementation. Good choice. However after six weeks of being on his program, well so I believed, he came to see me to tell me that what I had prescribed did not work. This can happen sometimes and my approach needs a bit of tweaking. Although I knew what supplements Murray was on, I asked him to remind me what he was taking and at what dose (as I do with my clients, be warned if you consult with me!). I was just checking. Can you see where this is going my friend? It turned out that Murray had not taken what I had prescribed or as I had prescribed it. Nor had he followed the diet exactly. For many days during the previous six weeks he had 'forgotten ' to take the supplements, or had left the house without them, or had only taken one a day. Supplements are not a 'quick fix', they are something that need to be taken on a regular basis in order for them to build in your system. Then, providing they are the right ones, they will work for you. Murray left my room with his tail between his legs, although we did manage to laugh about it! All alone in the pretty little pots, the supplements are of no help to the cause! Just like the glass of water I poured myself half an hour ago will not quench my thirst left sparkling in the glass in the kitchen! Silly Big Bird!

Invest in your health, but be wise, and make it an investment that counts. Like with everything, you get what you pay for and very cheap supplements could well be a purchase to avoid. However, even like fine wine, it is not always the most expensive on offer either that gives the greatest satisfaction. Quality rules. Eating a varied diet is always the best way to provide the body with the essential nutrients required to live a healthy life, but topping up your nutrient levels with potent supplements can make an even bigger difference in the quality of your health!

It's not the End, it's just the Beautiful Beginning......

'No need to run and hide, it's a wonderful, wonderful life.'
— Name that tune!

So here you are, my friend, you have reached the final chapter of The Wellbeing Touch book. Well done! But, this is only the beginning and certainly not the end, as although this book is full of great information, reading the book alone is not going to take you to a whole new level of wellbeing! (Sorry to drop that one in.) Reading this is the starting point of an exciting journey that maybe you need to embark on, one that sees you spring into action and implement any necessary changes to enhance your life. I am confident that I have given you uncomplicated foundations on which to build and hope that I have managed to inspire and motivate your journey too. I want you, and wish you, to be able to live an absolutely incredible, disease free, happy life. Now it is over to you!

This is your life so live each and every moment the best way you can (which is all we can ever do) so you can look back and say, 'Wow! What a wonderful, wonderful life!' See all the incredible things you have around you and practise gratitude for what you have. Take time to make the most of each day of your life, no matter what it consists of! Remember the present moment is a gift. Grab life by the horns and give it a good shake - so to speak!

In my humble opinion, (as if you had not worked this out) health is the most important part of your existence that you need to take special care of. Your health is vital to all aspects of your life and keeping it in tip top condition will play a crucial role in helping to determine how your life will be. Let this slip and your body and mind will pay consequences which may result in your whole existence being more of a struggle, more painful and less enjoyable. And why would you want that? Preventing disease is so much easier than curing it. It is the best course of medicine you will ever take and you do not need to visit the doctor to get a prescription for it! Learning to listen and work with your body, not against it, will bring dividends. Remember your body is your very best friend and not your enemy, so go with the flow. Feed your body the correct fuel and give it the right messages and hopefully you will dance through life with a constant spring in your step and a beaming smile on your face.

Listen to what your body tells you. If you are not feeling 'quite right', your body is telling you something needs to change, something is wrong. If you have continual stomach cramps, headaches, indigestion, sore throats or aching limbs, or you are constantly tired (which is a major complaint these days), this is a sign, or rather a huge red flag that is being waved at you! Take heed, rather than brush it off, put it down to old age, or make excuses that you are too busy. Like any open wound left in dirty conditions, it will fester, become infected, be the cause of general ill health and one day, maybe, even death. Don't risk that my friend! Sit down quietly and draw your focus to where there is an issue. Then decide how you will resolve it and most importantly, take action to do something about it in a helpful way....(flash back to Ernie and Bert here! You did read the Stress chapter didn't you? Just checking!)

You are powerful and mighty my friend, especially when it comes down to having control over your health. You are in the driving seat and setting the direction of your life. You alone are selecting the good or the bad, the healthy or the unhealthy, the fat or the thin, the tired or the boundless energy! Step up and choose the greatest of all the options. (If you were to give it some thought, you would not meaningfully choose the worst option would you?) So take the time to think first about what you are doing. Be your very own leading inspiration, your own guru of all things great, your own Super Hero (with or without the blue pants over the tights!).

It is time to give up blaming those around you for your present state or past mistakes, and instead take responsibility for yourself. If you do not like any part of your life, you can change it once you take responsibility. Whatever your beginning, and wherever you are now, you have the power to make the rest of your life incredible. All you need to do is decide what it is you want to change and then plan how you will do it. Then it is action stations, again! (Woman of action me, in case you have not noticed!)

Remember the saying, 'If you keep on doing what you have always done, you will keep on getting what you have always got!' If something is not working for you, please, don't be like so many others and tell us this is what you have done for years....because that may be so, but it is so obvious to the rest of us that - it is not working! If it is not working, you need to change the way you are doing it. Yes, change can be scary because it involves you stepping out of your comfort zone..... but you can do it! After all, do you really want to live all your life sitting in the same box? Don't just think outside the box, step outside it too.

See yourself as the incredibly gorgeous human being you are and fall madly, deeply, and passionately in love with yourself. Love all of yourself, even the cranky bits, the spare tyre, and the mind that forgets what you went upstairs for! Put your arms around it all and give it one humongous hug and tell it with sincere energy, that you love yourself. Your body is your bow, your heart your arrow. Be your own Cupid and aim for your soul! (Cheesy I know....but with a little work, great for a Valentine's greeting!)

Be who you are with conviction and have faith and belief in who you are. Stand in front of a mirror, hairbrush in hand, and belt out the song 'I am, what I am.' Boy will it will give you a dose of power when you need it!!! Everyone is awesome in their- own way and deserves that recognition, especially their own recognition.

Now, my friend, make sure your seat is in the upright position, your lap tray folded away and hand luggage neatly placed under the seat of the person in front of you (shoes off too for a more comfy ride). Remember the rules of flying - in case of an emergency, place your own oxygen mask on, BEFORE helping others. Look after number one first and then you will be in a far better position to look after numbers two, three and four! Indulge yourself in plenty of self-care. Spend time every day doing something, no matter how small, to make yourself feel special. Look after your skin, your nails, your hair and your appearance. Dress in clothes that make you feel good and let the reflection to the outside world be one of utmost self -respect. Be proud of who you are, you wonderful human being you! You owe it to yourself, and to the world as a whole to take the very best care of yourself.

There is far more to gain in life by being a creator rather than a competitor. Strive each day to create your life in the way you want it to be. Forget what others have, how they look and how they are, this is your life and so it is all about you. Leave others to their life. Don't waste your energies thinking about what the next door neighbours have that you don't. Instead invest your energy in you and create everything you want your life to be, step by step, slowly, but surely. Do not try to rush a good thing. First make something wonderful of today, for it is all you have in your hands to work with. Making good today will give tomorrow a great starting point. Move on from yesterday, the day before that and even the previous years... they have all come and gone and had their day. If I can do this, so can you! And I have and I do, hence so can you!

Next time you are at the checkout in the garage, or the supermarket, just for a laugh, ask for a top up of happiness. Go on, have some fun. I am pretty sure there will just be a vacant response of 'ergh?' But let me know if anyone offers you one! Remember you cannot 'get' happiness from anywhere, or have it taken away. It is a feeling, your feeling. If it is an external factor that is causing a less than happy state, change it. If you can't change it, then make life more pleasant and change your attitude towards it. Feed yourself happy stories, thoughts, and make laughter part of your daily routine. Have a bit of side-splitting fun. Create your own happiness as only you can!

There are a great many foods that feed feelings of misery, like sugar, processed foods, and fast foods. Make a plan to eat 'happy' foods, the foods that will work with the serotonin in your brain and help you feel happy which includes the luscious chocolate....just keep it dark and rich. Feast away on vegetables, whole grains, fruits, beans, lentils, nuts, free range eggs and quality meat and fish. Remember your state of mind will have direct implications on your health – it's all in this body mind connection that we experts harp on about! (Have I not done this!?)

Smile every day. Hold your head up, put your shoulders back, breath coolly, calmly and evenly, and spend a few minutes whenever you can practising breathing. I know it sounds a wee bit strange to practise breathing, but the more you become aware of it rather than just expecting it to happen, the calmer and more in control you will be, plus your brain will get an extra hit of cell-powering oxygen. You will be think much more clearly afterwards!

When people ask you how you are, do your best not to give them a miserable list of all your complaints. For one thing, it will not help you feel any better reminding yourself of all the things that are causing you grief. There is also nothing worse than to be on the receiving end of someone's varicose vein trouble or piles.......of undealt with financial affairs. It's enough to bring down anyone's day. Instead behave in a positive manner, inspiring others to do the same along the way. I am sure you would agree, because now you are an aspiring positive person, that it is far more pleasant to answer the question of 'how are you?' - by saying ' I am fabulous and life is marvellous, thank you!' As well as inspiring for some, it could also be quite annoying for those who are considered not such good friends to hear you on such fine form! He, he he!!! You will be surprised how lifted you will feel after and the shock may just be enough to get your conversation buddy to act in the same way! You never know, you may lift someone else as well as yourself, which is a kindness. I did this in the local supermarket the other day, when the cashier asked me how life was and I managed to stop him in his tracks (am sure he was waiting for a list of all things bad so he could add in all his woes) by telling him life is amazing. What's more, I had the whole queue behind me deciding this was the way to be! It was infectious, just like a smile! And I bounced out of the supermarket like I had won the lottery rather than having bought a bottle of water.

Why be so serious!? I mean, seriously! Of course there are times when you need to have your serious face on, but let it go when you can. Life is light, not heavy, unless you choose to make it that way. You do not have to be constantly serious, you can enjoy a more humorous approach to all things sent your way and life will come up a notch or two. Find amusement in

YOU and how you are! Give your head a shake like Donald Duck does, complete with cheek wobbling vocals, to loosen the seriousness. Start laughing at just how serious you are being. Think of your most serious face – got to be worth a giggle! You have the choice to spend your life being serious – in which case you need to have a serious think about the frown lines – or to spend your life seeing the lighter side. Relax, be playful, have an open mind - all of which can really lift your soul.

Follow the rules of stress management my friend, and get your stress under control. Remember there is no stressor on this planet worth ill health. Get hold of that piece of play dough and splat it! Yes! Feels so good! Recognise stress, step back, ground it, down size it, take control over it, balance it and act upon it in a beneficial way (Ernie and Bert. Have to ask you, do you get a picture of the Sesame street characters Ernie and Bert each time I mention the names? It could be quite good to see these every time you are stressed …..just to remind you how to be and maybe bring a smile too!). Do your best not to worry and be anxious as it solves nothing but often creates something else for you to worry over, which you really do not need. Instead face head on what is bothering you and draw up a plan of action (to infinity and beyond!) that will see things resolved. Then, my friend, you can kick your shoes off and enjoy this life which is a pretty darn fab way to go!

If there is any part of you worth some extra tender loving care, it is your digestive system. When it gives you a sign that it is struggling, stand up and listen (even if it is not making windy noises). It could mean the start of something more serious if left untreated. Nurture it with good food, a proper eating programme and boost your army of friendly bacteria. These guys ensure you have a supply of B vitamins, which, amongst other important tasks, will fill you with energy. Find out if you have a food intolerance going on, or if your digestive enzymes are not to their full quota. Whatever you do, don't treat your digestive system as a garbage deposit. Feed it and nourish it so it can do an optimum job of looking after you. My dear friend, I urge you to read the chapter on the digestive system again and again until you understand the importance of this astounding system, how it works and what it does to keep you well. It is the centre of your immunity, protect it in every way you can, so it can protect your life in return. Think of yourself as Leonidas, the king and protector of your people, keeping yourself well from your head to your toes and all that is in between.

Eat a balanced diet, full of the goodies that nature intended for us - fresh fruit and vegetables, nuts, seeds, beans, lentils, whole grains, eggs and quality meat and fish. Be inventive and creative with your food, and after giving your cupboards a detox, ban the processed food industry from entering them! Take a decision to enrich your health rather than line the pockets of the manufacturers of the most destructive foodstuffs on earth! You are one step ahead of their cunning plan now. At the end of the day it is exactly that uncomplicated to eat well – no processed foods, and plenty of what nature intended. Simple isn't it!?

Knock up a taste sensation in your kitchen and discover the hidden Jamie Oliver or Nigella Lawson (or mix of both) deep within you. You too can toss in the herbs and spices, whilst looking delicious yourself, and enhance the flavour of your new, healthy cuisine. And, as a result, benefit from the highest antioxidant levels around which are found in herbs and spices. These antioxidants will help to protect you, and your family, from the nasty invaders such as cancer and as an added bonus (buy one get one free!) they will also keep you looking young and beautiful. Create a little herb patch in your garden or decorate your windowsill with pretty pots full of fresh herbs. If you do not consider yourself to have 'green fingers' hang a lovely spice rack close to your cooker so it is easy to shimmy and shake a bit of spice into your food. You are the next Master Chef. What? You didn't know that?

When I am in Crete I love to see the way Greek families spend hours over a meal (that wonderful Mediterranean diet). It is always an occasion. Food should be a social event to be savoured and enjoyed, so aim to sit down and share it with friends and family. Eat slowly, chewing your food mindfully while enjoying the taste. Forget eating on the run as this impairs your digestion and is bad for you (along with the breakfast biscuit bar – which is no healthier than any other biscuit-designed for you to eat whilst running - frantically in the morning – awful things). Always stop to eat and give yourself time out whilst you do. Mealtime is an excellent excuse to have a little 'me' time.

They say variety is the spice of life, and never has it been more salient than in the case of the food you eat. The greater the variety and the greater the quality, the more diverse the nutrient content will be - although you do not need to load ten different varieties on your plate each mealtime as I have known people to do! You have all week to vary your food so stick to two or three varieties at each mealtime so as not to challenge your digestion too much. It is often the food you eat day in day out that will, in the end, be the cause of food intolerance, as your body becomes fed up of dealing with it. It is, there-fore, more beneficial on all levels to keep your digestive system surprised by a varied diet rather than the same old, same old!

We need a variety of nutrients to feed every cell and organ in our body, so that they may do their job of keeping you alive and well whilst you are, but it is best to go organic. It is a clever idea to cut back a little on portion size, which most of us could do with anyway, to be able to afford to eat organic. Wash your fruit and vegetables in water and cider vinegar before eating to cleanse away any chemicals, peeling skins too on occasions to ensure less chemical impact. Love the food you eat and eat the food that loves you!

What happens when you forget to water your plants? Sadly, no longer will they produce beautiful flowers for you to enjoy, but they will go a bit crispy, shrivel up and eventually die. Water is a life force without which you too will dry up like an old prune - not particularly attractive - and eventually die, even less attractive! You are like one huge walking puddle, remember, and your levels need to be topped up each and every day. Welcome the morning with a glass of water to hydrate your body from the very beginning, and wish yourself a good night with another glass to keep you hydrated through the long night. In between, here is the motto: 'sip away, throughout your day.'

Get out there and move it! Work that bootiful body and help it work for you. Raise your heart beat, challenge your muscles and get yourself a kick- ass rear view! Get out of bed and have a good old stretch. Crank up the volume of and sing along to 'I've got the moves like Jagger' and shake your little tush in the bathroom! Have fun and games with friends and family in the name of exercise. Leave the office and go for a walk in the air. Stand up and move around and stand for a while whilst working. Play like a child, join a club, a class, a gym, a team, and go for it! Remember to squat, lunge, push, pull and lift whenever you can. We humans were born to walk and walk we should as often as we possibly can. Just as we were designed to walk, we were also not designed to be static for hours on end and this is not conducive to a healthy disposition. So move every hour, walk around, be a bit irritating to the other half and fidget, stand up instead of sitting, whatever you can do to move your body, do it.

Treat yourself to a treatment plan or booster plan of supplements. Get well using a natural alternative rather than turning to medicine every single time. Practise forward thinking and boost your supplies before a certain time may deplete your reserves. Supplements are nature's nutrients in a convenient, high dosage form. Taking a supplement is merely enhancing what you should have naturally and, yes, you could probably do with one! Choose quality over price, or you could be wasting your money and putting more unhelpful substances into your system. Read the labels. Ask for advice from a professional like myself. Take your supplements alongside a healthy diet so you will truly benefit from your efforts.

You are not expected to know all you need to know about staying fit, healthy and disease free, not even after reading this amazing little book! Although, of course, I hope you are now somewhat better equipped. Nor are you expected to know how to fix things if they have gone wrong. Think about it, if your car broke down, you would not begin to fix it alone (unless you have been trained to do so). You would more than likely call the breakdown service and have a nice mechanic sort it all out for you. I know if I was to waste many hours under the bonnet of my car, I would probably make matters a whole lot worse! There are those out there who are trained to be of assistance to you in the field of health, both mental and physical. It is their job to offer you advice, treatment and answers. You are entitled to all of this as much as the next person, but you have to take the first step and go forward to get what you need. You have a responsibility to yourself, to take control over your life and the means to take action. Put a plan together. Fear nothing my friend, for way too much of what we fear never comes to pass. Whatever life sends your way, face it head on, be strong, determined and clever…. and deal with it.

At the end of all this, remember maintaining great health is not a complicated matter, unless you choose to make it so, and why would you do that? It can be as easy as eating a healthy, balanced diet, taking some daily exercise, adopting a positive outlook, practicing good stress management and supplementing with nature's medicine if you need to. And if you are in the unfortunate position that your health is currently challenged, remember nature has an awesome medicine cabinet at your disposal. Make the very most of what is on offer and boost your immune system every way you can and make a strong, determined bid to regain good health

You are special my friend, as unique as your DNA, a marvellous feat of ingenuity, and your life is your very precious gift. You hold it in your hands so keep it close, treat it well and never let it go. x

Acknowledgements

This is the part of the book where I am allowed to act like I have reached the top of my performance career and I give, with a little drama and the odd tear, my thanks as I collect MY Oscar!

I am a writer with very large 'L' plates attached to me, so I would like to give the greatest heart -felt thanks to my editor, Dr Catherine Maria Brusten, whose continual support, unbelievable patience,   gentle guidance and smart editing skills I would not have been able to get past 'go' without. The very lovely Dr Catherine, known to me as Kate, is also a much treasured and wonderful friend. P.S. I did not send Kate these acknowledgements for editing! (Thank goodness for spell check is all I can say! The grammar is Wendy Langley's unique style!)

I would like to thank my parents, who have just celebrated their 59th wedding anniversary, for getting it together and having me in the first place! Because of their amazing parenting skills, love and continual support throughout my life, I have got thus far and have been able to help, inspire and motivate many others on my way. Way to go mum and dad!

I would like to thank my two beautiful sons, James and Miles, who have filled me with happiness and pride as they have grown into handsome, intelligent, and kind-hearted young men. Being educated in the age of computers, they have been in the very fortunate position to be able to help mum when the computer is playing up, or more precisely, when I do not understand what I am doing or what I have done! Plus

Miles kindly instructed me on word (showing me how to put information in little boxes, which I am now a genius at, as you will see) and James has designed the wonderful cover of this book. Proud mummy moment!

I would also like to thank my son in law, Richard, for breaking his leg and hence having time on his hands to give his invaluable help formatting this book and launching it onto Amazon! There is always a silver lining to any situation my friend! And just to prove that there is nothing you cannot do if you really want to do it - just seven months after breaking his leg in two places, Richard completed his first half marathon, a distance of 21.1km in a time of 1:52:45. Get your running shoes on my friend!

I would like to thank my other half, who is lovingly known as 'The Resident Chef', for his patience with the hours I have ignored him whilst I have been having 'an affair' as he puts it, with my computer. Of course, the plus side of my work - it gave him extra time in the kitchen so he could muster up more delicious food! (See what I mean about silver linings?)

I would like to thank the beautiful island of Crete for the stunning locations I have been lucky enough to sit at, and be inspired by, whilst I have been writing (and tan topping!). Plus of course, all the little bars and cafés (and their lovely staff) who have supplied me with endless coffee, cool water and occasional wine!

I would like to thank all those who came into my life to teach me lessons, however horrible you were, so that I may grow and learn and then turn all my knowledge into a skill to help others.

I would like to thank all my lovely clients for their trust in my ability to help them through their challenging times.

I would like to thank you, my friend, for choosing to read this. I hope from my heart it serves its purpose and helps you.

And finally, I would like to thank my beautiful dog, Sugar and my five cats, Lucky, Africa, Mara, Sunshine and Snowy for their listening skills. Their acknowledgement is well deserved for it was their unfortunate job to listen to me read this book out loud, over and over again, from the very dodgy first draft, to the final read through - and they never complained once! They surely love the hands that feed them! Extra treats tonight girls!

www.ingramcontent.com/pod-product-compliance
Lightning Source LLC
Chambersburg PA
CBHW070636290526
45790CB00001B/110